Considered Choices

The new genetics, prenatal testing and people
with learning disabilities

Linda Ward
Norah Fry Research Centre
University of Bristol

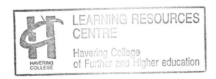
British Institute of Learning Disabilities

For Oliver Russell
In recognition of his longstanding commitment to the Norah
Fry Research Centre and to the pursuit of better lives for
people with learning difficulties

A free accessible leaflet on difference and choice for
people with learning disabilities is available from BILD,
tel 01562 850251

British Library Cataloguing in Publications Data
A CIP record for this book is available from the Public Library

ISBN 1 902519 62 0

© Copyright 2001 BILD Publications

BILD Publications is the publishing office of:
British Institute of Learning Disabilities
Wolverhampton Road
Kidderminster
Worcestershire
United Kingdom
DY10 3PP

Telephone: 01562 850251
Fax: 01562 851970
E-mail: bild@bild.demon.co.uk

Please contact BILD for a free publications catalogue listing BILD books, training materials
and journals.

BILD publications are distributed worldwide by
Plymbridge Distributors
Plymbridge House
Estover Road
Plymouth
United Kingdom
PL6 7PZ

Telephone: 01752 202301
Fax: 01752 202333

Contents

Acknowledgements

Thanks are due to the following for their help and support in facilitating the organisation of the original conference for which most of the papers included here were produced, and enabling the transformation of those – and other – papers into this book:

- Margaret Macadam, former colleague at the Norah Fry Research Centre, who bore the lion's share of the work involved in organising the conference;

- Oliver Russell, former Director of the Norah Fry Research Centre, for finding sources of financial support to enable us to spend some time working in this new area;

- the University of Bristol for the award of a Benjamin Meaker Visiting Professorship to enable Dr Marcia Rioux, then Executive Director of the Roeher Institute, York University, Toronto, Canada to spend some time at the Norah Fry Research Centre and contribute both to the conference and to our thinking;

- the former Special Trustees of the United Bristol Hospitals for funding towards the costs of the conference;

- the Margaret Egelton Fund for help with some of the costs associated with editing the papers for this book and bringing it to eventual fruition;

- Jackie Rodgers and Joyce Howarth for their commitment and creativity in working out how people with learning difficulties could be actively involved in the debate about prenatal testing;

- Alison Collins, Graham Hamblett, Zara May, Bruce Webster, Brenda Cook, Collette Harris and Jackie Long and their supporters for their participation in the two workshops which preceded the conference and to the first four of these for their powerful presentation at the conference itself;

- John Harris at the British Institute of Learning Disabilities for his continued commitment to the publication of this book and his patience despite repeated delays;

- Linda Holley at the Norah Fry Research Centre for her secretarial support;

- and, finally, all the people who helped us find a path through to some understanding of this complex and often inaccessible area, including those who contributed to the original conference, whether as presenters or participants.

Linda Ward
Director
Norah Fry Research Centre
University of Bristol
January 2001

Foreword

Tom Shakespeare

As I write these words, the world is waiting for the announcement of the outline map of the human genome.[1] By the time you read this, we will have a snapshot of the genetic makeup of the human species. It is obvious why this is so exciting for biologists, and for those of us who are interested in science. It is a genuine milestone in the development of planet Earth.

But this excitement should be put in perspective. First, we don't know what all these genes do yet. We don't even know how many genes there are: estimates vary from 30,000 to 150,000. The genome snapshot is a bit blurred. Second, genes are not the whole picture. After all, we share 98% of our genetic material with chimpanzees. We even share 51% of our genetic material with yeast! But there's obviously a big difference between us and these other life forms. The genome is not the meaning of life. Nor is it the blueprint for life. At best, it is a recipe for creating and maintaining a life form. As with every recipe, a whole range of factors affects the result. Different cooks, different ingredients, different ovens will produce very different meals.

People get carried away with the miracle of genetic information. But we should consider very carefully how to use this information. The discovery of the gene for Huntington's Disease was a mixed blessing. Knowing if you might become ill, and when you might die, is a frightening prospect. In practice, it has been found that only about 12% of vulnerable people wanted to find out if they carried the Huntington's gene.

---

1. Explanations of technical terms used in this book are given in the Glossary at the end.

Understanding genetics enables scientists to understand diseases and, potentially, to develop therapies and drugs to alleviate conditions. In the future, this will lead to better treatment for cancers, hypertension and a range of everyday problems. When there is no treatment for a disease, the major application of genetics will be in prenatal testing and selective termination of pregnancy.

But these practices need to be introduced gradually, and with extreme caution. I support a woman's right to choose whether to get pregnant or continue a pregnancy, but I am concerned about the context in which choices are made. Social information about what it is like to be disabled – particularly information from disabled people themselves and their families – is as important in making these choices as genetic or clinical information.

Reducing suffering and preventing impairment are goals that most people would support. But in our focus on genes and diseases, we should not ignore people and relationships. Disability is a fact of life. The human population is different in all sorts of ways; we should preserve diversity and recognise the moral value of every individual. Non-disabled people fear impairment. Disability is regarded as a medical tragedy, which should be avoided at all costs. Yet disabled people can enjoy a good quality of life, in a society which promotes more independent living and civil rights. Disabled people's voices need to be heard in genetics debates, including the voices of people with learning difficulties.

Fear of impairment was the trigger for eugenics programmes in the early twentieth century. The focus of eugenics was on preventing particular groups of people from reproducing, and on maintaining 'the quality of the race'. In the early twenty first century, we are entering a brave new world. The concern today is not so much about who reproduces, but who is to be born. While supporting individual choice, we should campaign to ensure that these decisions are not dominated by fear of impairment, or by economics. Cost-benefit analysis often drives the introduction of population screening programmes. Profit motivates biotechnology corporations who market genetic tests and interventions.

But these are not the most appropriate guides to drive developments in this complex area.

Understanding genetics requires difficult balancing acts. For example, only 1% of births are affected by congenital impairment, while 12% of the population are disabled. This indicates that environmental factors, lifestyles and ageing are the major causes of impairment, rather than genetics. Yet four in ten of us will develop cancer, and cancer is a genetic disease. We need to put genetic knowledge in appropriate perspective. Don't believe the hype, but don't believe the hysteria either. Our priority must remain to remove the barriers, in order to build a more accepting and a more inclusive world. Genetics will affect all of our lives. We need to understand how this might happen, and the nature of the social and ethical decisions we shall have to make, individually and collectively. This collection of papers will contribute to that process of learning and empowerment, and is to be warmly welcomed.

Newcastle
June 2000

1. To be or not to be . . .

Linda Ward

Introduction

Some years ago I received a letter from Marcia Rioux, then President of the Roeher Institute – Canada's national institute for the study of public policy affecting disabled people – which is renowned for its applied research on human rights, social inclusion and social justice.

She had become involved, through her activities with the International League of Societies for People with Mental Handicap (now renamed Inclusion International) in debates around the importance of the Human Genome Project (the project which aimed to map all genetic material contained within human beings) for people with learning difficulties.

She, and other colleagues, had become concerned at the potential negative consequences for people with learning difficulties and other disabled people of the Human Genome Project. These included the possibilities that people who did not have a 'normal' genetic makeup might be seen as less desirable, and that increasing use of prenatal testing and other new reproductive technologies might increase the pressure on parents to selectively terminate pregnancies where the foetus was, or was thought likely to be, affected by a 'disabling' condition. As a representative of Inclusion International on the International Bioethics Committee on the Human Genome Project of UNESCO she was writing to seek the support and involvement of colleagues at the Norah Fry Research Centre at the University of Bristol in raising awareness of these issues and carrying out research in this area.

Back then, in the early 1990s, I knew nothing of the Human Genome Project. At that time, press coverage of the Human Genome Project in particular and the new genetics more generally was limited (Durant et al, 1996). Accordingly, I wrote back that, at the Norah Fry Research Centre where I was employed, we undertook social, applied research. We were not scientists; how could we be involved in a subject of this kind? This book proves just how wrong I was.

A few years passed and press coverage of the Human Genome Project and other developments in the new genetics and reproductive technologies increased. But I still felt ill-informed on the issues and unclear about the relationship between these developments and our own social research on supporting people with learning difficulties more generally.

Then, I had the opportunity to attend an international seminar in Helsinki on precisely this theme. The potential negative consequences of this new science suddenly became clear. Contributors talked about the use of genetic information to discriminate against disabled people in employment, health and life insurance and a whole range of other areas (cf. Billings et al, 1992). I realised that sometimes science was too important to be left to scientists alone.

Fortunately, an opportunity arose to invite Marcia Rioux over to the UK to spend a few weeks with us at the Norah Fry Research Centre. We seized the chance. We spent time talking with her and learning more about the issues. We realised that developments in the new genetics had enormous potential consequences for disabled people and society generally. We also realised that this was a debate in which the voices of those most likely to be at risk of the adverse consequences of the new technology – that is, disabled people and those involved with them – were those that were least likely to be heard. Indeed, we could find, at that stage, no instances where people with learning difficulties had been involved in this debate.

We decided to organise a national event in Bristol to bring together a wide variety of individuals and organisations with a range of interests, expertise, experiences and views to contribute to this debate. We would call it an 'Information Exchange' because we wished to make it clear that while we valued the contributions of those labelled 'experts' in this arena, the views and experiences of those with a personal perspective on the subject were important too. As newcomers to this area at that stage we wrote to those people whom we knew from our contacts were regarded as the 'experts' in this field. We were amazed at their response. People were supportive and encouraging of our plan and keen to participate. And so the event (entitled 'Considered Choices?') was organised and took place with great success.

Having assembled such a rich range of contributors and participants for the event, and knowing of no other initiatives in this area relating to people with learning difficulties, we felt committed to ensuring that the contributions made on that day should be available for a wider audience. For a variety of reasons transforming those papers into this volume was subject to repeated delays, but returning to the papers afresh, after a gap of two years, it was clear that their contents were still topical. Indeed, with the increased public interest in cloning, genetically modified foods and the Human Genome Project generally, and the recent Consultation Report on prenatal genetic testing more specifically (Advisory Committee on Genetic Testing, 2000) they were, if anything, more topical than ever. So we decided to proceed with publication of most of the papers (some modified and updated) together with a new paper written for a special symposium on the subject at the Inclusion International conference in The Hague in 1998 and revised for this volume.

Contents

When we were putting together the programme for the Information Exchange, we were keen to ensure the participation of people with learning difficulties in the debate on a subject of critical importance to them and their families. We could find no examples of where this had happened before and were uncertain about how to proceed. Was it even possible to involve people who might, by definition, have difficulty understanding abstract concepts like 'genes' when even those of us without a 'learning difficulty' label sometimes struggled for under-standing in this area? Luckily, we had colleagues with commitment, confidence and creativity who were happy to work through the complexities involved in making accessible information and issues that were usually quite the reverse.

Chapter 2 of the book provides an illuminating account of the processes followed by Jackie Rodgers and Joyce Howarth in bringing together a group of people with learning difficulties on two separate occasions to consider what prenatal testing and the new genetics might mean for them.

Chapter 3 provides a detailed description of the workshops they organised and was put together by Joyce and Jackie with contributions from Alison Collins, Brenda Cook, Graham Hamblett, Collette Harris, Jackie Long, Zara May and Bruce Webster. Its title 'Difference and choice' encapsulates very clearly some of the critical issues at the heart of the new genetics debate. Undoubtedly, their input into the Information Exchange was the most powerful contribution of that day.

If prenatal testing and the use of genetic information raises profound issues for people with learning difficulties, so it does for their parents or prospective parents too. We are grateful to Sue and John Picton for their honest and open account in **chapter 4** of 'What it [prenatal testing] means for us', as parents of two young adults both with multiple impairments (caused by an undiagnosed, but presumed recessive genetic metabolic 'error').

Some of the issues involved in safeguarding genetic diversity while respecting parents' rights to choose are discussed in more detail in Oliver Russell's subsequent chapter (**chapter 5**) on this subject: 'Supporting families to make informed decisions', based on his experience both as a clinician and a teacher of medical students.

Priscilla Alderson's contribution (**chapter 6**), significantly entitled 'Unanswered questions', looks in more detail at the many questions raised by prenatal screening: Why we do it? Why does it makes women anxious? How can pregnant woman get better information?

It is only recently that disabled people have begun to demand some involvement in debates about the new genetics (see, for example Disabled People's International, 1998; Disability Tribune 2000). Agnes Fletcher, herself someone with an inherited condition, outlines graphically in **chapter 7** some of the dangers of the new genetics in relation to disabled people in the context of the history of eugenics, current pressures on parents during prenatal testing and the cultural pressures affecting choice, when the birth of a disabled infant 'is seen as nothing other than a tragedy for the family and for that child'.

Prenatal testing and diagnosis raise a huge number of ethical issues. These are coherently articulated by Ruth Chadwick in **chapter 8** 'Whose choice? Whose responsibility? Ethical issues in prenatal diagnosis and learning disability'. Unfortunately, the concerns of ethicists are seldom paramount in these debates. There are many others with different kinds of interests in this area. They include scientists, those with commercial and economic interests in research and development in genetics, lawyers, genetic counsellors, policy-makers and of course social scientists – as well as disability rights and other advocates for individuals and groups vulnerable to the implications of the new genetic research.

Marcia Rioux's paper (**chapter 9**) 'The many interests in genetic knowledge' brings an international perspective on prenatal testing and the use of genetic information in relation to people with learning difficulties which illustrates the huge vested interests active here.

Ethics, social inclusion and human rights
Perhaps the biggest change since we organised the original event on prenatal testing and people with learning difficulties back in 1997 has been the huge increase in public awareness – and indeed suspicion – about some of the risks associated with developments in genetic technology since then.

Public doubts about genetically modified crops caught politicians, farmers and food retailers alike by surprise. Assumptions about the presumed safety of new scientific interventions have been shaken by recent events, like the death of Jessie Gelsinger, an eighteen-year-old volunteer from Arizona, who died during trials of an experimental gene-based medical treatment in September 1999. He was the first person to die as a direct result of gene therapy, which had hitherto been hailed as a potential cure for scores of incurable diseases. Subsequent investigations arising from his death have uncovered multiple, and alarming, examples of unethical practice (for example, no evidence that patients recruited for the trial had been fully informed of the risks beforehand – Meek, 2000a).

There is mounting concern at the race by research and development companies operating in the area of the new genetics to patent genes, or at least the data of gene sequences, and perhaps seek a monopoly on tests to screen people for genetic disposition to certain conditions or diseases (Meek, 2000c). There is also concern at the insistence of some companies that publication of any information arising from their work (information which might transform some areas of medical research) be delayed for years in order to prevent commercial rivals from using it (Martinson, 2000).

There are worries too about the uses to which genetic information may be put and the potential discrimination against disabled people which may ensue. These worries led to the recent formation of the London-based Campaign Against Human Genetic Engineering (Meek, 2000b) and the establishment of the Human Genetics Commission to investigate the potential for discrimination by employers, insurance companies and so on (*Independent on Sunday*, 2000). A recent survey carried out by the UK disability organisation RADAR found that nine out of ten people thought it should be illegal for employers and insurance companies to have access to the results of genetic tests for fear that the information could be misused to refuse people insurance (Fletcher, 1999).

At the same time, there is concern amongst some disability groups that even where doctors may be relatively well versed in the *medical* side of disabling conditions, they know very little about the experience of living with them. Thus pregnant women may not receive the most accurate information when they undergo prenatal testing and may be unduly encouraged (even pressurised, some would say) into ending their pregnancies (cf. Dodds, 1997).

At a time when the British Government talks of trying to end 'social exclusion' and a Disability Rights Commission has been established in London to help outlaw discrimination on the grounds of disability, the need to be vigilant about the use and abuse of new reproductive technology and the acquisition of genetic information (to ensure its use does not increase discrimination against disabled people) becomes ever clearer.

This is by no means a straightforward issue on which disabled people are themselves united. Indeed, it is an issue on which there are strong divisions (*Disability Now*, 2000). Some see some of the possibilities promised by the new genetics, like 'gene therapy' as a potentially positive development (Association of Cystic Fibrosis Adults, 2000; Cystic Fibrosis Trust, 2000); many are acutely aware of the potential negatives involved (see Fletcher, chapter 7 this volume). And different individuals will have their own personal views about the difficult balance to be struck between upholding 'a woman's right to choose' to continue a pregnancy and the foetus' 'right to life' (see, for example, Bailey, 1996). These are indeed complicated issues warranting detailed analysis and debate and ones that do not offer simple, quick fix, solutions.

Prenatal testing and the new genetics may, as a respected public health doctor informed me recently, be 'public health' issues, but for many of us concerned about the rights of disabled people they are, more importantly, issues of ethics, social justice and human rights. We know that many of the disadvantages experienced by disabled people in our society are *not* a product of their impairment but of the poverty, negative attitudes, discrimination and disabling barriers in the society in which they live. We know that disabling conditions are not always, even mostly, the product of genetic 'disorders' alone, but are frequently a product of the interplay between genetics and the environments in which people live and their experiences. Indeed, if we were serious about reducing impairments, then we might do well to look at the social and the environmental factors so commonly involved (see, for example, Williams, 1997). If we truly wish to strive for a better and healthier society, then we will need to look beyond the genes of disabled people themselves to achieve this:

> *People with learning difficulties are different to other people. We get picked on – others make fun of us. People shout at us in the street sometimes. Black people with learning difficulties get picked*

on even more. People with learning difficulties should be treated fairly and not discriminated against. Scientists should find the gene that makes people pick on those who are different. Then our lives would be better.

(Participant with learning difficulties at 'Difference and Choice' workshop, chapter 3, this volume)

References

Advisory Committee on Genetic Testing/Human Genetics Commission (2000) *Prenatal Genetic Testing: report for consultation.* London: Department of Health.

Association of Cystic Fibrosis Adults, UK (2000) *Response to the Consultation Document on Preimplantation Genetic Diagnosis produced by the Human Fertilisation and Embryology Authority and the Advisory Committee on Genetic Testing, November 1999.* London: ACFA.

Bailey, R. (1996) Prenatal testing and the prevention of impairment: a woman's right to choose? In J. Morris (ed.): *Encounters with strangers: feminism and disability.* London: The Women's Press.

Billings, P.R., Kohn, M.A., de Cuevas, M., Beckwith, J., Alper, J.S. Natowicz, M.R. (1992) Discrimination as a consequence of genetic testing. *American Journal of Human Genetics*, 50, 476–482.

Cystic Fibrosis Trust (2000) *Consultation Document on Preimplantation Genetic Testing. Response from the Cystic Fibrosis Trust.* London: Cystic Fibrosis Trust.

Disability Now (2000) Much ado about genetics, May 1.

Disability Tribune (2000) Solihull Bioethics Declaration, March, 4–5.

Disabled People's International (1998) *Bioethics and Disabled People: Proceedings of a Seminar.* London: Disabled People's International, European Region.

Dodds, R. (1997) *The stress of tests in pregnancy*. London: National Childbirth Trust.

Durant, J., Hansen, A. and Bauer, M. (1996) Public understanding of the new genetics. In T Marteau, and M. Richards (eds.) *The troubled helix: social and psychological implications of the new human genetics*. Cambridge: Cambridge University Press.

Fletcher, A (1999) *Genes are us? Attitudes to genetics and disability*. London: RADAR.

Independent on Sunday (2000) Watchdog to tackle genetic discrimination, July 2, 8.

Martinson, J. (2000) Protocol on gene research at risk as firm demands exclusive rights, *The Guardian*, March 7, 3.

Meek, J. (2000a) Death exposes risks of gene therapy, *The Guardian*, January 24, 3.

Meek, J. (2000b) Ethical dilemma in race to map genes, *The Guardian*, June 15, 1–2.

Meek, J. (2000c) Patenting our genes, *The Guardian, Special Supplement*, The story of life. The mapping of the human genome, June 16, 8–9.

Williams, C. (1997) *Terminus Brain: the environmental threats to human intelligence*. London: Cassell.

Acknowledgement

Thanks to the Inclusion International seminar in The Hague, 1997, for the chapter title.

2. Difference and choice:

helping people with learning difficulties to consider ethical issues around genetics

Jackie Rodgers and Joyce Howarth

This paper describes our experience of providing training to help a group of people with learning difficulties to consider ethical issues relating to the use of genetic information to inform choices around pregnancy. We discuss how we approached the many ethical dilemmas we faced in the course of preparing and offering the training, and the effect that the work had on our own beliefs and values. We explain the strategies and safeguards we used to try and ensure that the people who came to the training got the maximum benefit from it. Finally, we consider the potential for future work in this area.

The ethics of providing the training

Before we approached people to see if they were interested in learning more about genetics, we had to give careful thought to the ethics of what we proposed to do. The least sympathetic explanation of this would be that we were undertaking a piece of research to find out what some people with learning difficulties thought about genetics, to increase our knowledge, imposing an agenda upon the people concerned and giving potentially upsetting information with no obvious benefit to them.

However, this interpretation was far from our intention. We shared a belief that people with learning difficulties have a right to information, and that it was not only reasonable, but desirable, to give them a chance to take part in a wider debate which was particularly relevant to them. The opinions of people with learning difficulties about developments in genetics had barely been addressed, and their voices seldom heard. Discussions about whether people with learning difficulties' lives are 'worth living' (Morris, 1991) were being made with little reference to the people who could surely offer the most informed opinions.

To engage in this debate, people with learning difficulties would need information presented in accessible formats specially geared to their needs. They would be less able to contribute to events such as the planned Information Exchange (the papers from which form the core of this book) if they did not have appropriate information beforehand. We wanted to offer training which would begin to meet such a need. Such an approach could be criticised for being impairment specific. However, the idea was not to separate people with learning difficulties from other disabled people or from anyone else engaging in the debate, but to allow them to participate on a more equal basis, with the help of appropriate preparation beforehand. This was no more impairment specific than providing a hearing loop to enable someone with a hearing impairment to take part in discussions.

While agreeing that it was valuable to give people with learning difficulties the opportunity to find out more about genetics, there were elements of the 'least sympathetic' interpretation of what we were doing that we wished to safeguard against. We recognised that while the genetics debate is of relevance to people with learning difficulties generally, it would not necessarily be of interest to every individual. If we were to avoid 'imposing an agenda' upon anyone, it was important to ensure that anyone who took part did so through their own interest and with informed choice. We had to ensure that the main reason for giving people the opportunity to take part was to fulfil their own interest in gaining more information about the topic, and that an opportunity to take part in the general Information Exchange would be an optional extra. We also had to acknowledge that the information we would impart was potentially upsetting. It was likely to include matters which were new to the people concerned, which could highlight the existence of a widely accepted world view which was essentially hostile to them. We were therefore anxious to include certain safeguards in our approach to finding people who wished to take part, and to the training generally, which we will go on to describe in more detail.

Challenging our values
When planning the training we intended to focus on the same issues as the general Information Exchange: the use of genetic information to inform choices around pregnancy. This was a key issue, of relevance to

people with learning difficulties; the training should enable anyone who wished to take part in the general day to be better prepared to do so. When we began to prepare the programme we both found we began to question beliefs and values we had held over many years.

We would both describe ourselves as feminists and strongly supported a woman's legal right to choose on abortion. However, these beliefs did not sit easily with support for a disability rights perspective that a foetus should not be aborted solely on the grounds that it has an impairment. A woman may exercise her 'right to choose' specifically because an impairment is diagnosed or suspected. The medical and legal systems privilege this choice by allowing abortion on the grounds of 'severe handicap' until the time of birth, rather than the usual 24-week limit. There is no definition of what constitutes 'severe handicap', and there is no way of knowing the severity or mildness of learning difficulties associated with, for example, Down's syndrome, before birth. There is also the question of whether the abortion of a foetus on such grounds is ever right, however profound its impairment.

We both spent time together and apart trying to find a way forward with these conflicting beliefs, at times finding ourselves examining belief systems around a 'right to life' which had previously been anathema to us. After many headaches and cries of 'ethical dilemma break', we found we could move forward by acknowledging the validity of both views, and respecting the position of anyone who chose to follow one or the other.

We, ourselves, ended up acknowledging both views simultaneously. This was not a comfortable position, but one which met our individual needs through the course of the work and which recognised the complexity of the issues we were tackling.

Originally we had planned to work with a co-facilitator with learning difficulties in carrying out the training, as we are both committed to the inclusion of service users in work which relates to them. We had one day planned into our preparation time to go through the programme with the person concerned. However, the person we had hoped to work with was unable to make the course dates. With hindsight we felt that this was fortunate. It became clear that any co-facilitator would need to go through the same process as us, of thinking through their thoughts and values, as well as possibly needing to find out more about pregnancy and reproduction generally. We had not allowed sufficient time for this, and we realised that to involve a person with learning difficulties as co-facilitator when they had not had such an opportunity would have been a tokenistic and unprofessional approach.

This experience reinforced the message that involving people with learning difficulties in training means involving them from the outset, in all planning meetings. They need to be supported to work through whatever the issues are for themselves, whatever the subject area. This was yet another ethical dilemma we had to face, since we believe in involving service users in issues that concern them, but felt it would not be appropriate in this situation. We did feel, however, that the people who came to the course could be regarded as potential co-facilitators for future work in this area, as they would have had some opportunity to think through the issues in the way that we had done.

Maximising benefits and minimising any potential ill-effects
Our initial approach to finding people who wished to take part was to establish for ourselves who the training was for. We were aware that what we were offering was new and that there was little previous work to draw on to work out the most appropriate and helpful approach. We thought that a fairly small, intimate group would be best. This would allow people to get to know each other better and to share their feelings more easily. Within a small group, we hoped to have space for people with a variety of backgrounds and experiences. We wished to include both men and women, thinking that there might be gender specific issues to explore. We decided that we were not aiming the training at people with any particular genetic condition, but that the debate was of relevance to all people with learning difficulties. So, although the group, which eventually met, did include some people who had particular genetic conditions, they had not been invited specifically because of this. Since the work was new to us, we were not confident of our abilities to make the issues accessible to people with profound intellectual impairments, and the course that we devised was most suitable for people who had moderate learning difficulties.

Our initial thoughts about what would be included in the two days available suggested that some discussion of reproduction, pregnancy and abortion would be needed. This would be to help people understand the basic meaning of 'genetics' and learn about testing in pregnancy and the choices available to people. We were both aware, not least because of previous work about people with learning difficulties' knowledge and awareness of sex (Howarth, 1995), that many people would never have had the opportunity to learn even basic information about sex and reproduction. We did not feel that the two days' training would be an appropriate or sufficient format to educate people for the first time on such matters.

We therefore decided that the training we would offer would be aimed at people who had some prior knowledge of sex and reproduction. While this seemed the correct, if pragmatic, approach at the time, it did leave us concerned that we were excluding people who might be interested, but who did not have such knowledge. It also left us with the difficult practical issue of finding out whether people had such knowledge beforehand. With the benefit of hindsight we know now that the technical details of what 'genetics' is and how testing in pregnancy is carried out were not essential for people to understand the debate about genetic information and choices in pregnancy. However, we did need to discuss abortion, and there is little doubt that the prior knowledge of the people in the group we worked with enabled them to gain a more detailed understanding of this debate. Having undertaken this work, we now feel it might be possible in future to design training for people who do not necessarily have such prior knowledge, which would still give them some access to the debate about genetics, prenatal testing and abortion.

We decided it would be most appropriate to offer this pilot training to people who were in supportive environments. This was to help ensure that people had someone on hand subsequently to discuss any difficult issues as they thought of them and after the training had finished. We got in touch with people through informal networks, using our own knowledge of supportive environments locally. We also decided it would not be appropriate to approach anyone who was experiencing any sort of acutely stressful situation at the time, since exploring the issues raised for the first time might involve its own stresses, which might be unwelcome to anyone already having personal difficulties.

As another safeguard we visited each person who might be interested in taking part personally, before the training, to fully explain the programme and allow them to make an informed choice about whether to participate. This discussion included the question of who would be available to offer them support, both on the day if they wished, and afterwards. It also gave us a chance to explain more about the training to supporters in the person's life and to discuss any of their concerns or interests.

In these ways, we established a range of strategies before the training took place, aimed at maximising what people would gain from it, and minimising any potential negative effects. We also ensured that a pocket of money was available if the matters discussed brought to the surface deep and uncomfortable feelings for anyone who took part that meant they would benefit from short term professional help, beyond that which could be offered by their supporters. In addition, we identified the type of resources that were available locally if it seemed anyone might benefit from longer-term help and counselling. At times we felt that we were perhaps a little over-cautious in the attention we gave these matters. However, we were aware that what we were offering was new, and there was little previous work available to indicate how people with learning difficulties might react to exploring such issues. It therefore seemed better to have a full range of strategies in place in case they were needed, while at the same time not approaching the training as if it was so sensitive and difficult that the need for such help would be inevitable.

On top of the particular strategies described above, we worked at creating a supportive environment in which the training could take place. In choosing a venue we looked for somewhere warm and welcoming, which was fully accessible for disabled people and also accessible geographically. We ensured that transport was available to suit the needs of the individual, involving them in as little hassle as possible and paid for from our budget. Recognising that meal and drinks breaks would play an important part in the days, we discussed the sort of food that people liked with them beforehand and responded to particular tastes in what we offered. Everyone who came along valued such attention to detail. The food provided was rated very highly in the evaluation, being given two large stickers when one large sticker meant excellent!

Our aim of creating a supportive atmosphere to explore the issues seemed to be fulfilled. The supporters who accompanied people played a key part in this. We had previously given supporters some brief written guidance about their role. This emphasised that their main task was to offer practical and emotional support rather than to participate. It also identified that discussions around the topics we were to address could raise difficult issues for supporters as well as participants, and that they would need to consider this when deciding whether to agree to accompany someone, and to think about whom they could discuss *their* feelings with.

We were pleased that when people did choose to bring along a supporter, those that came were very good at their job. They worked with appropriate sensitivity and involvement both with the specific individuals they accompanied and with others in the group. We were also gratified by the support that the people who participated gave each other. People were helped through difficult moments by their peers and there were several plans to continue friendships after the event.

The process of devising and presenting the training held many difficult, as well as satisfying, moments for us. Support for the trainers was essential. This was partly gained through supporting each other. Our experience suggests that work of this nature would be much harder for anyone to undertake alone. It was also helpful to be working alongside colleagues at the Norah Fry Research Centre who were struggling with similar issues. More formal strategies in the form of supervision and debriefing were also important. Finally, we felt very supported by the people who attended the training and the supporters who came with them. It felt much more like a mutual exploration of difficult issues than a didactic teaching process.

Finding ways to explain the issues

We found it very beneficial that we had had the opportunity to think and feel through issues that were very difficult for us, before we planned the materials for the course. To give people attending a similar chance to work through all the complex issues we were presenting, we needed to work through them ourselves first. Only then could we give them the space and unbiased information they needed. We think that it was inevitable that our values still came through, but they did so less strongly than they would have done if we had not gone through this process first. They became one view among others that could be respected, rather than any sort of definitive 'right' set of opinions.

While planning the two days, we were unable to find any resources to help explain ideas and issues which might have been new to people. It was a challenge to find concrete and accessible ways to explain things such as 'abortion', 'genes' and 'genetics' and 'prenatal testing' or 'screening'. We found that we had to gain a good understanding of these areas ourselves before we could begin to find accessible explanations. The help of Marcia Rioux – who has been actively involved in work around genetics and people with learning difficulties internationally (see chapter 9) and who was in the UK at the Norah Fry Research Centre at the time – was invaluable in both ideas and support. Subsequent editions of the popular soap opera 'Eastenders' (BBC TV), in which a character had to decide whether to go ahead and have a baby that would be affected by spina bifida, would have been a useful resource. Perhaps videoed excerpts could be used in future training.

We felt that it would be helpful to explain 'genes' in terms of what makes people different from each other. During the course we spent time thinking about how people in the group were different from each other. This led to looking at how these differences came about: for example, through people's preferences, their culture, how much money people have got, whether they experience discrimination, and finally through their genes. We then looked at the fact that there are laws that say that some differences should not be taken into account in areas such as employment, and that differences are okay – they are just differences.

From here we looked at how a foetus is formed, with the sperm and egg meeting, and explained that on each there are pieces of information that fit together, called genes. The genes have information for things like what you look like and what illnesses you might get. We talked about things that 'run in the family' and people then drew what they thought might be 'on' some of their own genes. There was discussion about whether people's learning difficulties belonged 'on their genes' and it was recognised that sometimes they did and sometimes they did not. This led on to talking about how doctors might find out if a baby would have learning difficulties before it was born. We found a video on prenatal care that had a short piece showing a woman having a scan, which was useful and offered another medium for sharing information.

It would have been all too easy to present a particular view on abortion, simply through the materials we used to explain it. For example 'right to life' campaigners make use of very explicit images of a foetus developing in the womb, depicting it as much like a baby as possible, while 'right to choose' activists tend to emphasise an image of the foetus as small and like 'a bunch of cells'. We searched for ways of explaining abortion and the present law relating to it in as balanced a way as possible. We decided to bypass both sets of images by presenting pregnancy as time passing, from January through to October, using an illustration which showed the passing of the seasons over 40 weeks. We could then identify the different stages where the law allowed abortion on the grounds of 'severe handicap' and where it was allowed in most other circumstances.

We felt that it would be helpful to explain abortion in terms of making choices about whether to have the baby you were pregnant with. Time was spent looking at the choices people made in their lives. This provoked mixed reactions, as some people were very happy with the choices available to them while others were angry at the lack of choice they experienced. This helped when the group began to examine why people might choose to have an abortion. We explained that if someone decided they did not want to have a baby, they could have an operation that would stop the baby growing. After giving information and discussing issues about abortion, it was important to allow people time to explore what they felt about it all. We did this by running a continuum, allowing people to choose where to stand in the room from the extremes of 'feel good' at one end to 'feel bad' at the other. We had successfully used this method the previous day to explore how people felt about their lives and found it a good way of allowing people to express their feelings even where they were less able to do this verbally. This exercise helped people realise, and hopefully accept, that everyone had their own feelings and views.

For some participants thinking about abortion raised strong emotions that needed sensitive handling. This was one stage where the value of having two facilitators was shown. One facilitator could work with someone who was upset, while the other worked with the group. However, we also realised at this stage the strength of support available within the group. Everyone showed how they felt for one particular individual's pain around this, and one participant stayed to help support that person while the rest of the group carried on working. The individual concerned later said that this peer support helped a great deal.

Some of the methods we used were adapted from other training; some were new to us. The methods used seemed to be successful, as people joined in the discussions and sessions received positive evaluations at the end. A few concepts (for example abortion) needed explaining several times for some people, partly we think because of their potentially disturbing implications.

Conclusions
The process of devising and offering this training was challenging and thought-provoking but satisfying too. It had a considerable emotional impact upon us. It not only made us question values and beliefs that were important to us, but also brought home the personal impact of the oppression faced by people with learning difficulties. It made us realise the breadth and depth of opinions that people with learning difficulties have to contribute to the debate around the use of genetic information. It helped us to understand that what seem to be very complex issues can be explained to people with learning difficulties if a sensitive and creative approach is employed. It made us think that people generally can contribute far more to the debate if it is not presented as the province of knowledgeable 'experts'.

The work we undertook felt like a beginning, with a huge amount of possible future work ahead. Accessible resources are needed to enable people with learning difficulties to understand concepts such as abortion, genetics, screening, as these issues very much affect them. The work here was done with people with moderate learning difficulties, but work also needs to be aimed at people with more severe learning difficulties over a longer period of time. Funding needs to be committed to such work, as it is vital that people's voices are heard on these issues.

At the heart of any future work there must be far more sexual health awareness and information for people with learning difficulties. It is often assumed that people with learning difficulties' understanding of current debates around genetics is limited by their intellectual capacities. We believe it is frustrated far more by a widespread lack of access to basic knowledge about sex and reproduction. This does not necessarily require further funding; what is needed is staff who are willing and able to talk about sexual matters with the people they work with. Support in this work can be found through other agencies such as health promotion services. This knowledge would allow people with learning difficulties to gain a much fuller understanding of genetics and abortion, enabling them to have greater access to a debate that has repercussions on the way that society as a whole values them and welcomes them into ordinary life.

References

Howarth, J. (1995) *The SHARP Report*. Bristol: Bristol Area Specialist Health Promotion Service.

Morris, J. (1991) *Pride against prejudice: transforming attitudes to disability*. London: Women's Press.

3. Difference and choice:

a workshop for people with learning difficulties

Joyce Howarth and Jackie Rodgers with Alison Collins, Brenda Cook, Graham Hamblett, Collette Harris, Jackie Long, Zara May and Bruce Webster

This chapter is about discussions and activities that took place during a two day workshop for people with learning difficulties on issues surrounding the use of genetic information to inform choices around pregnancy. The workshop programmes are reproduced at the end of this chapter.

Day 1: Friday 13th June

10.30 am Tea and coffee

People began arriving from 10 am. Taxis had been arranged, to try to ensure there would be no problem in getting to the venue. Seven people with learning difficulties were due, with three supporters. Everyone had been visited by Joyce or Jackie, so knew someone there and everyone had gone through the programme, to help overcome initial nerves about what was going to happen. One man with learning difficulties didn't appear – phone calls to his home revealed that he had got the dates wrong and had gone out. The staff there sent out search parties, eventually found him and he arrived an hour late. This was a relief, as there was only one man present, which might have made him feel a bit isolated if the other man had not turned up.

Getting to know each other

People began to relax and realise that some of them had already met at different events; this led to catching up on lives and general gossip amongst everyone there, before we did the 'official' introductions. People introduced themselves by saying their name and where they were from; this also introduced everyone to the fact that one of the women had severe hearing loss so used British Sign Language to communicate and used an interpreter. This then led on to the cushion game – a cushion was thrown from one person to another, with the thrower saying their own name and the name of the person they were throwing to. It was fun, with the cushion flying all over the place, being caught and missed, and in the process everyone learnt everyone else's name.

Expectations

People were split into three groups, with a supporter in each group (a pattern followed for the rest of the two days) and asked to discuss and record on flipchart paper why they had come, what they hoped they would do and what they hoped they would learn. This generated a lot of discussion.

Group 1

We've come to talk about babies who haven't been born – all babies because they don't know what they have come into. Babies – whoever they are, whatever colour, black or white, should have a chance to come into this world.

We have rights to have a baby.

I want to learn a bit more about it, what comes out of the day. I want to get right into it – all the surroundings of it, understand more about it.

I want to talk about how babies should be treated. Babies are not for five minutes – they are for life, for bringing into this world with love and care and respect.

We'd like to share with people what we all think with people here today, and what we get out of it. About our feelings and expressions.

We do not want people to choose for us. We want to be able to meet to say what we want for our own selves. Without staff/management/parents/anyone interfering in every way. And they don't know what damage they've done and how it can make you suffer. We don't want to suffer in silence.

Group 2

Why we came: to learn about differences and choices – why we are all different, about things we discussed with Jackie and Joyce.

To learn about each other.

About what happens to women after they give birth.

Hope to do: listen to different people talk, have a nice lunch, know everyone here better, talk about what we thought of today, talk up and speak about ourselves and different experiences we all have.

Group 3

To learn more about how babies are born. Want to know more about sex and condoms, want to learn more about how my body works.

To think about relationships.

To think about the future and being with my boyfriend and marriage.

Thinking about my feelings.

Spend time in small groups, be able to talk in private.

Thinking about choosing who you spend your time with.

Ground rules

The whole group decided the following ground rules for the rest of the course together. Everyone seemed to understand what was needed here with little explanation required.

Talk one at a time
Put your hand up to talk
Listen to people
Not interrupt people

Don't talk too much
Keep the door shut
Keep things said private

This chapter would seem to negate the last ground rule. However, at the end of the course we discussed how other people could find out what was discussed and everyone agreed it could be written up from the flipchart sheets as long as no one was identified. One woman also wanted some personal things she had said to be excluded, so we went through the sheets together and marked them to make sure they were not included.

My life as a person with learning difficulties
In three different groups, people were asked to list or draw on paper, with a supporter's help where needed:

- What I'm good at and what I like about me

- What others like about me

- What I like about my life, things I do, where I live and the people in my life

This was full of a whole variety of things and included being good at driving, looking nice, writing poetry, swimming, singing, signing, doing tapestry. One group wrote:

There are so many good things about our lives there isn't enough time to write it all down.

They were then asked to look at what they would like to change about themselves and about their lives. Every group included in this part that they would like people's attitudes towards them to be changed. Each person was asked to decide what would be the most important change for them; what would make most difference to their lives.

Change people's attitudes, not to be called mentally handicapped or other names. Stop people teasing. Like to show people what it is like to have learning difficulties – educate them.

Not just change Bristol's attitudes but make changes worldwide. Would mean people with learning difficulties can emigrate if they want.

It's difficult with people who don't sign, I can't talk to them, it makes me angry and sad. Why can't you sign?

I'd like to get married to my boyfriend.

I would like the lady I live with to listen to me and find time to talk to me.

Things to get better in my life – everything not to be so difficult.

Changing being hurt and used by other people.

Lunch
By this time everyone was hungry. Lunch was from Wholebaked Café – a café in Bristol in which people with learning difficulties work. Everyone helped to change the room round ready for eating. It was a relaxing time, with jokes, gossip and learning more about each other. One man was particularly interested in the signing and began to learn one or two words so that he could speak a little to the woman who used it to communicate.

How I feel about having learning difficulties
For the after lunch session we had decided to use a fairly active exercise to help people think about, and express their feelings on, their lives. This involved having two large signs, one with 'Feel good' and ticks, the other with 'Feel bad' and crosses. These were placed at either end of the room with an imaginary straight line between them. If anyone didn't want to take part, that was okay – they would not be asked to explain why. We chose statements people had written before lunch about their lives and asked everyone (supporters included) to stand on the part of the line that showed how they felt. After the first statement everyone got the hang of it. They were then asked if anyone wanted to say why they had stood where they were. Generally the people who stood at the 'Feel bad' end went there because of how they were treated by other people, not

because they felt bad about themselves. The people who stood in the middle for different statements often had very mixed feelings – for example, they felt okay about having a learning difficulty, but not about being called names in the street because of it.

What makes people different from each other

In groups, people were asked to list all the ways in which they were different from each other – it may have been how they looked, how they spoke, how they enjoyed spending time, where they lived. Supporters were asked to take part in this as well.

The lists were long and diverse, covering many aspects of appearance, ways of living and personality. All included learning difficulties and some specified Down's syndrome and Fragile X syndrome. One group wrote at the bottom of their list:

> *We shouldn't be any different because of learning difficulties or Down's syndrome – we're all human beings.*

We talked about how differences may come about – ideas which included culture, preferences, education, how much money people have, whether they experience discrimination, and genes.

It was when we moved on to looking at how people reacted to differences and to the participants that stories of prejudice, fear and oppression came out. One woman in the group was Afro-Caribbean, and she spoke of the way that others, particularly men, shouted things at her in the street, calling her a 'black bitch'. She was frightened and angered by this, not understanding why people wanted to upset and frighten her. She said they also shouted about her learning difficulty and it seemed unfair that there were two things that people used against her. The rest of the group were shocked by the racism but could empathise, as all of them had suffered in this way at some time in their lives – something it is easy for non-oppressed people to forget and hide from. There were also stories of the way professionals, and doctors in particular, had treated people unfairly or nastily because of their learning difficulty.

After everyone had had their opportunity to speak about this, we talked about the laws that were supposed to stop discrimination; people wanted to know why the laws were broken so much, and why disabled people weren't really protected. We also talked about the policies in many workplaces that try to ensure equal opportunities, but also how many places expect you to be able to read and write to be able to apply for a job, an area that equal opportunity policies rarely cover.

The final decision was that differences are okay – they are just differences.

A break was needed after all this!

Genes

The group had ideas about how other differences came about, but did not understand much about genes. We asked how a baby was made and someone talked about sperm and eggs meeting. We drew this on flipchart paper, to try to illustrate further for those who didn't know this part of reproduction. We explained that on each sperm and egg are pieces of information that fit together like a jigsaw puzzle; the information says something about what you are going to be like; they are called genes. In the large group we discussed what might be 'on' people's genes, and began to talk about things that 'run in the family' – for some this further explained the concept.

Participants were then asked to work in small groups and draw or list some of their genes. One person put:

My bones, my height, a woman, my looks, asthma, my hair.

Another included:

Smile, teeth, knees, hearing, eyes (blue), nose, height, brains.

Some people wanted to know if their learning difficulty was due to a gene. We explained that sometimes it is and then you might be able to find out if a baby is going to have a learning difficulty before it is born. Some thought that this was a good idea, as parents could then be ready for the birth and find things out that would help the baby.

Thinking about today
We ended by going round and everyone saying something that they had thought about during the day. A range of issues were mentioned and generally the comments were positive.

Day 2: Friday 20th June

10.30 am Tea and coffee
This was like welcoming back old friends – people caught up with what the others had been doing in the last week. Although there didn't seem to be a real need, we played the cushion game just to ensure that everyone could remember names. It was more fun than last time, as it was much easier to remember and use people's names.

Making choices
In the large group we talked about what sort of choices people made in their lives. This varied from what to eat, to where to live, to whether to get tipsy and where to go on holiday. Some choices people wanted to make – to marry their boyfriend, for example – they felt they were not allowed by family and/or staff. Some people had more choices available to them than others. In small groups, they were asked to draw a house and round it draw or write the things that helped them to choose – this may have included who they talked to, what sort of information they had, the sort of pressure they had to make a decision.

> I would like to choose to live with my boyfriend but I have no choice where to live or which centre [to go to].

> It was up to me. I was sad to leave old friends. It was different, there were more people around. Staff are there to help. I chose for myself. I'm happy.

> I went on holiday with people from the house before deciding. There was no pressure, I could take my time to decide.

All of this was shared in the large group and brought out a mixture of anger and resignation from those who felt they were not allowed to make choices and felt very unsupported in their lives.

At this point we had a well-earned break, as this session had been hard work and brought up different feelings for people.

Choices in pregnancy

We then talked about how when a woman is pregnant, the man and woman might sometimes decide not to have the baby; the woman could have an abortion, which is an operation to stop her being pregnant. For some people this was quite a new concept and needed to be gone over again in the large group. The supporters continued with this where necessary in the small groups, where participants were asked to discuss why people might make this decision and what sort of pressures there might be.

Some people found this very difficult, as they were trying to cope with a new concept and find reasons for it happening. It was quite painful and difficult for some to put themselves in the shoes of people who may not want a baby, especially if they wanted a child of their own and were being given definite messages that they would not have any. Other people, for whom this was not a new idea, came up with a list of reasons why people might decide they wanted an abortion, which was similar to a list many groups in society might come up with, including that the foetus might have Down's syndrome.

We moved on to the law on abortion, which everyone found fascinating, especially the fact that 'severely handicapped' foetuses could be aborted up to birth. We explained that the tests women have can show if a baby is going to have Down's syndrome and some other conditions such as spina bifida and achondraplasia (a condition which means people do not grow very tall). There was quite a lot of discussion on what was meant by 'severely handicapped' and whether that made it okay to have different laws. We explained that two doctors are needed to agree that you need an abortion and one woman commented:

> I don't understand. If you have thought about it and talked with your friends and supporters, why do you need two doctors to say you need an abortion?

The group had strong feelings around the whole issue of abortion and were pleased when we said we could all discuss it further after lunch.

Lunch

For different reasons we both left the room for a moment after announcing it was lunch time. When we came back in, every person was involved in a task to get the room ready. Apparently this was done without discussion – each person looked round, remembered what needed to be done and got on with it, as part of a team. At the same time there was much chatting and joking going on as well as checking out how others were feeling. This was one of the points that showed how well people had gelled as a group and how supportive and thoughtful everyone was.

Feelings and thoughts about abortion

As the continuum had gone well the previous week and it was a form that the group was now familiar with, we decided to use it again for this part of the programme. There was far more spread of opinion on this than there had been with the previous topics, so we reiterated that differences are okay, that it is very difficult sometimes to accept that someone else thinks differently from you, but it was just difference, not right or wrong. First the group, including supporters, was asked what they felt about foetal testing.

> *I feel that a scan is good, as it means you can see your baby otherwise it is better to wait for the baby to be born.*

> *Tests are good because they give people information. Information means that people can seek help from their GPs.*

Next they were asked what they felt about abortion. People were spread between the two points with small groups at either end of the room. When asked what took them to that place there were impassioned pleas for unborn children and a strong feeling abortion was bad from the 'Feels bad' end. At the 'Feels good' end there were very definite statements on choices being very important and this was another choice people should have. On abortion of a disabled foetus or one with a learning difficulty there was a range of opinions and feelings:

> *The foetus should be aborted if a test shows it has a learning difficulty because I don't think it should be born into a cruel world.*

Disabled babies are okay.

It is not the baby with learning difficulties that's the problem it is the way the baby may be treated by everyone else.

At this point one of the people in the group, who has Down's syndrome, began to cry and talk about how her mother would have aborted her if she had known before she was born. This distress was compounded by many other things in the woman's life – a lot of anger, fear and hopelessness coming through. She was clear later that she wanted this reported as she wanted people to know what it was like, hearing talk about aborting disabled foetuses, when they were talking about people like her. She felt lucky to be alive and despairing about aspects of her life. Two other women in the group particularly supported her in her distress, allowing her to talk and cry, and talking about the awful prejudice they had met in their lives. The rest of the group listened for a while; then it was appropriate to move on.

Next the group were asked to think about what might be useful for people who had been told their foetus was going to be disabled, when they were trying to decide whether to have an abortion.

A video of what people with learning difficulties can do.

The baby will have other people to help out when they are older.

Don't think of the baby as having a label – they will get treated differently. Think of the baby as a baby first.

The people in the group thought it very important that people with learning difficulties are involved in any future debate about the use of genetic information to inform choices in pregnancy. They thought this could be done by having conferences aimed at people with learning difficulties, as well as speaking at conferences aimed at medical and scientific professionals. Some people also thought a video or other easy to understand information for potential parents faced with decisions about the possible abortion of a foetus with learning difficulties would be useful, looking at what people can achieve and the lives people live.

Political action by both people with learning difficulties and their allies was thought to be another way forward.

After a much-needed break the group came back to start thinking about the Information Exchange seminar that was coming up. Four people decided they would like to speak at the seminar – the others already had something organised for the date it was on. The group as a whole decided what areas should be covered, and the speakers chose which area they wanted to speak about. The speeches were written with support at a later date, as time had run out. However, here is what was said:

Our achievements

I have Down's syndrome. Because I have Down's syndrome some people have treated me badly. People have called me names.

I can do lots of things and enjoy my life.

I can use buses.

I go to the cinema.

I have friends.

I take part in performing arts. I've performed in plays.

I paint and make things. A mask I made was in an exhibition this summer.

I have a learning difficulty but I learnt to drive. I took my driving test and have a full licence.

I have got the Duke of Edinburgh's Bronze Award. I had to find my way across the countryside with a group of people, using a map. We had to camp out as well.

People should not treat us differently. We can achieve a lot if we are given the chance.

Differences

Everyone is different but people shouldn't be teased just because they are different. Some differences we talked about are eye colour, hairstyles and colour, good tastes, skin colour, music tastes.

When I was at school, I knew a girl whose fingers and toes were stuck together. I was frightened of her because she looked different. My mum found out I was frightened and made me walk to school with her and her mum. I got to know her and we became friends, and I liked her. It is important to find out about the person, not the condition.

People with learning difficulties are different to other people. We get picked on – others make fun of us. People shout at us in the street sometimes. Black people with learning difficulties get picked on even more. People with learning difficulties should be treated fairly and not discriminated against. Scientists should find the gene that makes people pick on those who are different. Then our lives would be better.

The importance of choice

People should have the right to choose and to take responsibility for their actions. Everyone makes mistakes. I like choosing where I live, making choices in my home such as what I eat, what cleaning I do and choosing my furniture. It is important for people with learning difficulties to choose these things for themselves just as anyone else would. Not having choice makes people feel embarrassed, hurt, disappointed and angry.

We feel we should be allowed to make our own choices. We want to choose things like where we live, what work we do, if we want to go to college. I chose to live with deaf people. I have my own flat and I can sign and communicate with everyone.

Disabled babies

When a lady is pregnant – we talked about what if the baby is disabled or has learning difficulties. I think babies with learning difficulties or disabled are good, very, very good. They should be born, not aborted.

There should be tests for women who are pregnant, to see how the baby is. If it has Down's syndrome, the parents need someone to talk to. They need to find out what people with Down's syndrome can do. You should think of the baby as a baby first, not just that it has Down's syndrome.

All that was left now was to evaluate the course. Everyone had been given a programme before the workshop that was set out in symbols. The evaluation was done by giving everyone another copy of the programme and three different size stickers. A small sticker meant they did not like that session, a medium sticker that it was okay and a large sticker that it was good. Overall, the vast majority of the sessions were awarded large stickers. The final round, where everyone was asked to say one thing they felt about the two days, were very positive, including statements such as:

It's important we get a chance to talk about these things.

It was good to meet new people and learn new things.

They also talked about one thing they were looking forward to. And then everyone went home, leaving us elated, drained, humbled and impressed by what we had experienced.

Thinking about difference and choice
Programme

Day 1 Friday 13th June 1997

 10.30am   Tea and coffee

 Getting to know each other

 My life as a person with learning difficulties

 Lunch

 How I feel about having learning difficulties

 What makes people different from each other

 Finding out about differences before birth

 Thinking about today

 4.00pm   Home

Day 2 Friday 20th June 1997

  10.30am   Tea and coffee

                Welcome back

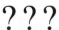   Making choices

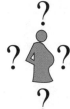   Choices in pregnancy

                Lunch

                How are we feeling/what are we thinking/what we want to do now

                Telling the doctor's conference what we think

                What I thought of the 2 days

  4.00pm   Home

4. What it means for us:

two parents' perspectives

Sue and John Picton

I. A mother's view

As a parent I have thought a lot about today and what I want to say. I am concerned that what follows is seen as personal, and to some extent not even a reflection of my husband's views (his comments come later) even though he is our daughter and son's father and my husband/partner. Other parents will have other views or opinions. I am not a practising Christian or follower of any religious faith; we live in a culturally diverse society, and I respect the right of people to have different views on major ethical issues. My husband is a practising Catholic; we have different views on the principle of abortion, and I certainly do not accept the Pope's teaching on birth control. Both issues are relevant to what I have to say.

Concentrating on and discussing the ethical issues is very important but every time I asked myself a question to write this paper, I either ended up with another question or, if I had an answer, it often appeared a contradiction of what I had just said or thought!

What is prenatal screening? What is it to be used for? What is this use of genetic information referred to? What is a learning difficulty?

Prenatal screening

Screening in the dictionary is defined as a) 'guarding from injury, danger or punishment' or b) 'examining systematically so as to separate into different groups'. This raises a number of questions for me. Are all pregnant women to be screened? What is the risk to baby and mother? How accurate are the tests? What conditions surround the screening? What genetic information is involved? What is this to be used for? What is it that we are guarding the unborn child from or what groups are we separating, and why? What is 'normal' anyway (screening implies some abnormality) and what is undesirable? How do we measure or evaluate the future life of an unborn child? There are many points of view as to what is desirable or undesirable for a successful life in our society today. Moreover, not all points of view can be accepted as having equal moral status. Medical intervention is creating huge ethical dilemmas. Many foetuses now continue to birth that would formerly have naturally aborted; many babies now survive that would previously have died; knowledge can now be obtained that was not available in the past. The ethical arguments today are inextricably caught up in the values of contemporary society – who and what is valued? And do we share any common values?

The term 'screening' seems to be used within the medical world in both senses of the definitions found in the dictionary. In today's context we are talking about tests being offered during pregnancy (prenatal). Screening today is more often than not used to inform a woman of the condition of her unborn baby. Has it got Down's syndrome? Has it got a disease, or some particular condition etc? In the majority of cases prenatal testing provides evidence for a termination of a pregnancy, although we are beginning to see treatments available prenatally for some medical conditions. However, if all prenatal screening led to treatment does this ease the ethical dilemmas? After all, it would then not lead to the very difficult and painful decisions about termination. (Whatever ethical stance is taken on termination, it is never easy, and it is not something that any woman positively seeks, particularly once they have conceived a child and are beyond the very earliest stage of pregnancy.)

If this screening is not to be used as a basis for a termination, or the option of one, is it to be used for a 'cure'? What of the dilemmas of identifying a condition like Huntington's chorea, which is late-onset and life-threatening, for which the medical profession can offer no help or treatment? What does this knowledge do to the quality of life of the individual concerned before the onset of the condition? Would they prefer to know or not to know? What are the risks to the baby and/or the parent of prenatal testing anyway? Is it intended, in fact, to exterminate those with undesirable conditions? What are undesirable conditions? Who makes these decisions? How are they made? There are huge ethical concerns here.

How does screening or prenatal testing address issues around the 'quality' of life or issues around tolerating and embracing difference? For example, even if all Down's syndrome babies could be 'cured', (along with other babies with other genetic conditions that appear to transgress what society deems 'normal') it still leaves terrible concerns for me as a parent. None of us knows what tomorrow will bring; we can become sick, have an accident, or perhaps develop some condition post-natally that leaves us 'disabled' in our current society. (I note also that it is estimated that 87% of disabled people are not born with their impairment.) If society expects all 'abnormalities' to be screened out prior to birth, how will it treat those who subsequently become disabled? People who are disabled are only just beginning to challenge the prejudice and discrimination that exists, but much remains to be done. Can prenatal testing and screening and the use of genetic information assist in the struggle for an end to discrimination and negative stereotyping for those in our society who are disabled?

What happens to those babies who escape the screening/testing process and are born and survive with conditions that are potentially screenable? What of their parents? No screening service is infallible. I used to privately yearn for prenatal screening and the option of a termination after we had produced Jo and Matthew. We wanted more children and in my role as a young mother, conditioned to expect a 'normal' child and unable to see how we could cope with a third child with a disability, I felt this would offer me the possibility of a child who would grow and develop 'normally'. I could also, twenty years ago, answer the almost inevitable question from those who met us – "Couldn't they [the medical profession] warn or tell you about your second child?" – that there was then no screening, that no one knew the cause, and they still don't. But the implication was that if we had known and continued the pregnancy we would have been irresponsible. We had produced 'drains' on society. Who was to bear the cost of their care? If those with the very best of intentions were provoked then to respond in such a way, as a parent I can see only that the situation is much worse for young parents today. And how much worse after eighteen years of Thatcherism with its emphasis on 'self-reliance', individualism, materialism and worth measured in economic productivity and so on? Prenatal screening and the use of genetic information can be used as a powerful political tool to promote fascist, selfish and inhuman materialistic values.

Termination or cure

But to return to the options that screening offers – my husband is a Catholic, and morally and ethically unable to accept termination. It would have wrecked our marriage. When I actually thought of the reality, rather than the idea of termination, I realised that I probably could not have gone through with it then, let alone in more recent years when my attitudes to disability have evolved with greater awareness of the issues involved. (That is not to say I believe there are never conditions or personal situations where termination is justified.) What value would it have given our existing children who were growing and developing in their own way if I had considered a termination of pregnancy subsequently? I just made sure I did not become pregnant again. What is a 'normal' child anyway? Many so called 'normal' children present or cause even greater grief, pain, anxiety and exhaustion than our two did.

If prenatal testing can only offer a termination as an outcome it may create a society where those born with a learning difficulty are accepted even less than they are today. (In any case, such testing cannot identify, let alone assess, many learning difficulties.) If it can offer a cure, without changing values and attitudes in society, it implies acceptance of a medical model of disability (that impairments need to be 'fixed') that is ethically unacceptable to me today. The medical model does not present a learning difficulty as just one of the many 'differences' that may exist between individuals in our society; or indicate that 'learning difficulties' is not an absolute condition but more a long continuum that embraces us all in some aspects of our lives. A 'social model' of disability, on the other hand, recognises that learning difficulties only 'disable' because of the attitudes, physical obstacles and emotional barriers that our current society creates. Nonetheless, I know that if I could still have children and was offered a cure for my unborn child I would accept it. Much as I love my daughter and son, and see them as individuals I feel I could not refuse such treatment. I wish I could have spared them the surgery and the negative responses of some people that they have had to endure. Where does this leave my ethics?

The medical world has already made enormous advances in understanding the workings of our brains and bodies. If medical science, by screening and the use of genetic information, can eradicate congenital conditions that lead to disabilities in our imperfect society is this not good? Does it matter whether this is achieved by termination or cure? In either case, it still leaves us, as parents, with terrible dilemmas and guilt about our innermost feelings. It also accords our children, of whatever age, a very questionable value. (Remember too, that society prefers young children with disabilities, and that our children's acceptance by society decreases as they grow to adulthood.)

Valuing diversity

We want our children, as they grow up, to be offered the dignity, choices and respect that is their right. When we are not around and cannot ensure they have this, who will? If screening and the use of genetic information is used to promote a 'super race', who defines that 'super race'? What will society do with those who are not of the 'super race'? There are enough problems already for those outside the mainstream of our society. Value too often is equated with wealth and the ability to fend in every way for yourself. Even if the 'perfect' child is born how will society ensure that perfection continues? We have to reverse the selfishness and lack of care for those who are too young, too old, too poor or too disabled to fend for themselves. Prenatal screening and the use of genetic information must be handled very carefully, within a framework of values that encompasses diversity, and values everyone.

We, as parents, have been lucky in many ways. Our children have not been very dependent on medical services. They are healthy and they do not need any specialised care. However, they are highly dependent in other ways and we have had huge problems finding appropriate adult provision for them. In many ways we still hope we can survive them, so we can make sure they do not suffer any neglect or abuse or indignity, that is all too often the experience of those who are dependent on others.

Prenatal screening and testing and the use of genetic information must not be used to fuel the forces in society that promote abortion as a 'solution' to disability, prejudice, discrimination and intolerance. During any debate on the value of these procedures, it is too easy for society to harden its negative attitudes towards people with learning difficulties. Many people are ignorant of what learning difficulties are. Too many assumptions are made about what people can, cannot or do not have a right to do. We need a massive programme of public education that informs society and challenges the negative stereotypes, prejudice and discrimination that exist.

What of adults with learning difficulties wanting a child? Every person and every case has to be considered individually. There are many parents without learning difficulties who abuse their children. My daughter is probably too disabled to bear a child, but what if she had been more able? Do we deny their rights to those who are able to bear children and enjoy sexual relationships? Where does prenatal testing come into this debate?

If prenatal testing is reduced to a cost-saving measure, as many reports in the media suggest is the case, I have very little hope for the future of our society today. We have to value difference, and accept that some people will need assistance, medical help, therapy and so on.

What does the future hold? Would we today be one of a 'blacklist' of parents who refused testing, or refused a termination? Modern information and communication systems are much more powerful and intrusive than they were when my children were young. Health care is already 'rationed' in some areas of medicine: what other sanctions will be developed for those challenging the majority opinion of medical professionals?

II. A father's view

No one wants their child to be disabled, yet the familiar images of 'tragedy' or 'disaster' do not and cannot help. The reality is that disability is central to what it means to be human. I honestly have no idea what Jo and Matthew think about being disabled; and given their communication difficulties I doubt if it would be helpful even to try and find out. On the other hand, they are happy and they bring happiness to others, including us, their parents, and this is work that really matters. So this is not some kind of dewy-eyed sentimentality, for living with them and making good their disabilities is very hard work. What is more, all sorts of things, for example, a conventional social life or the kind of level of professional work that would bring career advancement, do not and cannot happen. But I would not be without Jo or Matthew to save my life. They strip away pretence and ambition. They force me to face up to my own faults and limitations.

Who is to judge the value of another's life? Who has the right to say that a life is not worth living, that it should be squashed out? We exist for one another and, as a result, none of us has the freedom simply to do as we wish; we delude ourselves if we think otherwise. Rather, we have the duty to care for each other. That is the society I wish to be part of.

I do not see how any of us has the right to stand in judgement over the value (or the potential value) of the life of another, no matter how old or young or disabled. Time and time again I have listened to people (usually medical bureaucrats) say that prenatal testing and screening should be available as a matter of course to all pregnant women, accompanied by termination in the event of a diagnosis of disability, because it would be cheaper than the costs of looking after a disabled person. That is disgusting. On the other hand, I think we do have the duty to minimise the possibilities of disability in the life that has been created, for example through appropriate medical care (perhaps including prenatal screening and therapy) and through the avoidance of toxic substances.

We have created a world in which material gain, success, and choice seem to be the ultimate virtues, with little attention given to the substance of the choice that is made, or the manner in which success or gain are achieved. It is a matter of the kind of society we wish to create; and there are a great many moral questions and choices that transcend the immediate interests of the individual(s) concerned. In my view, this is the essential problem with the 'woman's right to choose' argument. I do not stand in judgement over anyone's right (including the right of a mother pregnant with a child diagnosed as disabled) to act in conscience within the law; but the law as it now stands permits the termination of a pregnancy for reason of the disability of the unborn child at any point within the full term of a pregnancy. I too have the right, within the law, to say that I do not believe this is right.

I repeat what I wrote at the beginning: it seems as if no one wants their child to be disabled, yet the images of 'tragedy' or 'disaster' do not really apply and cannot help. The reality is that disability is central to what it means to be human; and people can and should be supported through their disabilities and through their participation in the disabilities of others. Then, rather than dividing people into the 'able' and 'disabled', we can live and work together to make the kind of world in which everyone is valued for what they are. Jo and Matthew are important for what they are. The story begins here.

5. Supporting families to make informed decisions:

how can we safeguard genetic diversity while respecting parents' 'right to choose'?

Oliver Russell

Introduction

New genetic research now occupies a central place in the biological sciences. Modern research and technology raises questions about whether this knowledge is leading to a renewed eugenics movement. This paper is about rights and social equality:

> *With the possible exception of slavery, the genetic technologies represent the most profound challenge to cherished notions of social equality ever encountered.*

Mehlman and Botkin, 1998

Its concerns are the use and abuse of new technologies:

> *It has proved far easier for scientists to develop tests for genetic diseases than to devise effective interventions to prevent manifestations in people who are born affected.*

Holtzman and Shapiro, 1998

These matters evoke powerful feelings in all of us. Once we have stripped away the technical issues, we are faced with a very basic debate about whether we believe that some unborn infants can be said to have more value than others.

The debate is essentially about predicting the future. Advocates of the new genetic technologies claim that prenatal testing will enable doctors to predict which children will be born with a genetic or chromosomally determined disability, which children will develop such a disorder later in life and which children will be carriers of genetically determined disorders. They admit that the techniques cannot predict the quality of life that an individual will enjoy; the extent or effect of any impairments a person may have; or how a person may respond to the support, stimulation and affection which they may receive.

As Kitcher has commented:

> *Genetic tests cannot foresee the shapes that future people will give to their lives, thereby constructing the map that locates their central desires, much less anticipate the contingencies that will affect whether those desires are fulfilled or shattered.*

Kitcher, 1997

My perspective is that of a doctor who is involved in the teaching of medical students. For over 30 years I have been responsible for introducing student doctors to some of the ethical issues which are likely to affect them in their future practice as physicians. However I am not a philosopher, I am not an ethicist, and I am not a geneticist.

Making choices

Supporting families to make informed decisions about their unborn child is a daunting and humbling task. As a psychiatrist who is engaged in supporting and working with people who have learning disabilities, I work with people who carry a range of diagnostic labels – Down's syndrome, phenylketonuria, Sanfilippo syndrome, Fragile X syndrome – to name but a few. As a doctor I know something about the ways in which biological differences may affect the everyday lives of the people with whom I work. But more important to me as a psychiatrist are the emotional and environmental pressures which couples may face when making decisions that may have a profound impact on them and on the lives of others.

In my teaching I try to provide medical students with a framework to develop an understanding of how genetic technologies have an impact on the lives of families and individuals. Medical students will need this understanding if they are to develop an ethical and soundly based practice in their work with families. I focus on how we can support

families to make informed decisions when faced with prenatal testing –
and in particular to ask how we can safeguard genetic diversity while
respecting the parents' right to choose.

Do unborn infants who are different because they are found to have
abnormal chromosomes or who have genes that are associated with
developmental abnormalities count for less than unborn infants where
no such genetic difference has been identified ?

Disability, handicap and the social context
Marcia Rioux (1996) has referred to three critical factors in the
application of the new genetic technologies:

First, the assumption that disability is accounted for by an individual's
genetic makeup. She believes that this is a false premise that is based on
a false presumption:

> *Even were genetic diagnosis perfected so that it could be carried
> out early and non-invasively, it could never be effective in
> eliminating disability . . . more than 90 per cent of infant
> disability is because of social and not genetic causes.*

Rioux, 1996

Second, that disability is *a priori* an undesirable trait. The underlying
assumption is that there exists some social consensus or agreement
about what constitutes a 'perfect' baby. The idea of ensuring the
perfectly able-bodied, able-minded human is both an irrational and a
dangerously eugenic premise.

Third, that this simplistic equation of disability and individual genetic
composition obscures the enormously complicated set of factors that
result in disability and handicap.

> *Handicap is a social construct. If prevention of handicap is the
> real agenda, then an understanding of the material conditions that
> cause handicap must be seriously addressed.*

Rioux, 1996

I agree with Rioux up to a point. I agree that we do need to approach handicap as a social construct. I agree that the notion of the 'perfect baby' is irrational and dangerous. However, I believe that genetic factors are important and significant ingredients in human development that cannot be ignored. The new genetic technologies are here to stay and we have to face the fact that parents need to make decisions based on the best information available. Parents are forced to face painful and difficult decisions and doctors should assist them by providing the best possible predictions of what life may be like for their unborn child and of the supports which will be available to them.

Prenatal decisions and Down's syndrome
The couple who discover that their unborn child has an extra copy of chromosome 21 probably anticipate that their child will have a life which will be more limited than that of their brothers and sisters. But how will that child's life differ from that of their siblings? And how will that child be supported by the society in which they live?

Prenatal serum screening is now offered to 70% of pregnant women in the United Kingdom (Wald, Huttly, and Hennessy, 1999). But the situation facing parents who have been told that they have a high risk of having a Down's syndrome child is not clear cut. Twenty years ago, when amniocentesis first became available, many doctors and prospective parents treated the discovery of an extra chromosome 21 in a prenatal test as an automatic signal to proceed to a termination of the pregnancy, believing that the life of any child with Down's syndrome must be highly restricted. That is no longer the case. It is now appreciated that children and adults with Down's syndrome may grow up to have fulfilled lives, to enjoy companionship with others, perhaps even to have a job and a home of their own. Doctors can no longer advise parents that a child with Down's syndrome is destined to live a life in institutional care with few achievements and a poor quality of life. Of course, for some children and adults with Down's syndrome life may not be so good, opportunities to learn may be denied, and social isolation and rejection may be the norm.

Technological developments in recent years have made it possible to recognise that a developing foetus has the signs associated with Down's syndrome much earlier in the prenatal period than ever used to be the case. A new test, the nuchal translucency test, is reported to have a detection rate of 80% for Down's syndrome, and a rate of false positive results of 8% (Snijders et al, 1998). This is a non-invasive measurement based on the use of an ultrasound scan to measure the thickness of tissue at the base of the skull of the developing foetus. By combining the results of this test with the results of blood tests taken in the first trimester the rate of detection of Down's syndrome can be raised to 85% – with a false positive rate of only 0.9% (Wald, Watt and Hackshaw, 1999).

Women who are tested in pregnancy are forewarned that all tests carry some risk of error. For those who are screened and receive a false negative result – that is, where the results of the test were negative but they nevertheless deliver a Down's syndrome infant – we might expect there to be considerable psychological consequences.

But one recent retrospective study found that this was not the case (Hall, Bobrow, and Marteau, 2000). A sample of 179 parents of children with Down's syndrome was followed up for between two and six years. The study compared the adjustment of parents who received a false negative result on prenatal serum screening with that of parents not offered a test or who declined a test. The results of this study suggested that overall the parents in the sample had adjusted well to having a child with Down's syndrome. Levels of anxiety, depression, and parenting stress and attitudes toward their disabled child were similar to those in parents of unaffected children. But for some a false negative result on prenatal screening may have a small adverse effect on parental adjustment as much as four years after the birth of the child.

Many parents believe that with love, nurture, and support, people with Down's syndrome can enjoy a life of fulfilment, and defy the gloom and doom that used to lead some doctors to advocate abortion whenever the extra chromosome was found. Parents faced with the dilemma of making a choice may be prepared to provide love and care, but they can never be sure of the level of support that will be available from the community. For some parents it is a matter of economics: that they will not be able to pay for special help or programmes. For others, the problems stem from community attitudes which view 'Mongol' children as defective and to write them off at birth.

> *So, moved by concern for the future happiness of the child who would be born, they decide – reluctantly and against their deep commitments – to terminate the pregnancy.*

Kitcher, 1997

Tom Shakespeare, a powerful advocate of disability rights, suggests that there are nevertheless questions of degree at stake. He takes the view that few would oppose all screening and termination, just as few would support the promotion of widespread eugenics. He argues that between these extreme views there is a need for informed debate:

> *... and it is one which needs to take into account very many details and differences between people, pregnancies and impairments.*

Shakespeare, 1997

Clearly parents cannot make choices in a moral and social vacuum. Unless changes in social attitudes keep pace with the proliferation of new genetic tests, we can expect that in the future many prospective parents may feel they have to conform to social attitudes which they themselves may reject and resent:

> *They will have to choose abortion even though they believe that a more caring or less prejudiced society might have enabled the child who would have been born to lead a happy and fulfilling life.*

Kitcher, 1997

The decision to terminate a pregnancy in such circumstances is painful and difficult:

- parents carry the responsibility for making these decisions;
- society carries the responsibility for setting the social context in which these decisions are made;

- doctors, genetic counsellors and others will try to advise and support those who have to make these choices and live with the decisions they have made.

I suggest that we can recognise four models of decision-making among parents faced with the decision over whether to proceed with a prenatal test.

First, those who hold firm religious and moral views. Those who hold that sanctity of life is all-important will absolutely refuse to contemplate the termination of a pregnancy under any circumstances. These parents will defer to religious authority in making decisions or to their own moral principles.

Second, those who live in communities where state-enforced eugenic laws are applied and where decisions about the termination of a pregnancy follow the political directions of the state. Because of the political situation in which they find themselves these parents are not permitted to make their own decisions.

Third, those parents who are only able to contemplate having a perfect child and who will take no risk whatsoever that an unborn child might have a genetic disadvantage. They practise a personal form of eugenics that derives from their personal belief system.

Fourth, those who are in the middle of my spectrum. These are parents who are reluctant to destroy an unborn foetus, but who do not want to bring a child into the world who will suffer ill health, severe distress and serious disadvantage. They recognise that they may be faced with eugenic decisions but wish to make their decisions on grounds which they feel are ethical, based on the quality of life likely to be enjoyed by the as yet unborn child.

Social pressures may lead to families being blamed for making 'wrong' decisions:

> *The offer of termination of affected pregnancies will make us less tolerant as a society towards disability and difference and might*

*lead to blaming of parents who do not use genetic tests and
subsequently give birth to a child with a disability.*

Marteau and Croyle, 1998

Prenatal screening remains contentious because of the fine line between
allowing couples to make informed choices and pressurising them to
terminate the life of an affected foetus (Gill and Richards, 1998).

Eugenics

The decisions facing parents confronted with the results of prenatal
testing bring them face to face with the realities of eugenics. I believe
that eugenics is here to stay.

> *Eugenics seeks to respond to our convictions that it is
> irresponsible not to do what we can to prevent deep human
> suffering, yet it must face the challenge of showing that its claims
> about the values of human life are not the arrogant judgements of
> an elite group. If eugenics were simply a theoretical discipline
> there would be little fuss.*

Kitcher, 1997

Francis Galton (1892) introduced modern ideas on eugenics. He wanted
to apply the growing knowledge about human heredity to shape the
characteristics of future generations. Eugenics brings together the study
of heredity with some particular doctrines about the value of human
lives. We can all recognise that there is widespread concern about the
danger of a eugenic approach but perhaps the most basic objection to
eugenics is whether there is any system of human values that can
properly be brought to bear on decisions about genetic worth.

> *Genetic information used for negative purposes could undermine
> fundamental notions of social equality . . . Society risks becoming
> divided into those who are genetically sound and those who are
> genetically afflicted.*

Mehlman and Botkin, 1998

Kitcher (1997) believes that Western democracies practise 'laissez-faire eugenics'. Each parent or couple is free to make their own decisions. He sees the danger that we may retain the most disturbing aspect of past eugenics – the tendency to try to transform the population in a particular direction to reflect a set of social values. Unequal wealth is likely to result in unequal access to genetic information and to unequal opportunities to genetic screening.

Social support systems
Disabled people already fear that the spread of prenatal tests will erode the tenuous systems of social support that have made it possible for many people to go far beyond the limits once foreseen for them. If those social support systems decay, then prospective parents will experience an ever more relentless pressure to eliminate those whom their society views as 'defective'.

To be able to make their own decisions without external pressure, parents need to know not only how the genetic condition of the foetus may affect the life of the person to be born, but also that the society in which they and the child will live is committed to provide them with help and support. Only if prospective parents are assured that all people, however disabled, have a serious chance of receiving respect and support can they make a decision on the basis of their own values (Kitcher, 1997).

Making an informed choice in an ideal world
At the present time prenatal tests are not universally available. Those who have money, who belong to a health insurance scheme or who live in a country with a free national health services (as in the UK) will have access to tests. Those who are outside of a health care system are unable to gain access to prenatal testing. We may one day see a time when reliable genetic information from prenatal tests will be available equally to all citizens. Maybe there will be widespread public discussion of values and of the social consequences of individual decisions, but there should be no societally imposed restrictions on reproductive choices – citizens should be educated to make informed choices and not coerced. Finally, there should be universally shared respect for difference coupled

with a public commitment to realising the potential of all those who are born (Kitcher, 1997).

Protecting genetic diversity

We now recognise that our ability to detect genes greatly exceeds our understanding of what they actually do. Recent commentators have observed that even in disorders which affect only a single gene the relation between the DNA sequence of that gene and the bodily effects of that genetic change is far from clear. Genetic research and screening for genetic disorders have the potential for doing great amounts of good and great amounts of harm. We can anticipate that the way in which human societies move into this arena will be shaped as much by social forces as by concerns for the general 'public health' (Duster, 1990).

The future of the human species depends on our ability to maintain genetic diversity. I believe that there is a real danger that through the selective termination of genetically abnormal foetuses we may homogenise the human gene pool to such an extent that our species will lack the genetic diversity to respond to future environmental challenges (Mehlman and Botkin, 1998). This is a potentially serious problem. Indeed some genetic mutations, for example those associated with sickle cell anaemia and thalassaemia, may have reached their high population frequencies because the presence of the gene is associated with a greater resistance to malaria (Weatherall, 1991).

Conclusion

To return to my title: 'How can we support families to make informed decisions — how can we safeguard genetic diversity while respecting parents' right to choose?' I believe that we have to face up to the fact that the 'new genetics' is going to increase the pressure on many parents to seek the perfect child. Eugenic pressures are not going to go away. When a foetus has been diagnosed as having an impairment then parents have the right to know about alternatives to abortion, to learn about positive life perspectives for people with disabilities and assurance that they will have adequate access to necessary services and supports.

Pressures on parents to terminate pregnancies where the foetus has been found to have a genetic makeup related to a developmental disability will increase. Most doctors do not have sufficient information about disability to advise families about their choices. There is a need at such times for a disability advocate – a person with full information about the lives of disabled people who can play a role in ensuring that the decisions which are made are informed decisions (Roeher, 1998). Parents must be free to choose but they must be supported in that choice. We must ensure that parents are provided with better support, better information and an opportunity to decide, without being put under duress.

References

Duster, T. (1990) *Backdoor to Eugenics*. New York: Routledge.

Galton, F. (1892) *Hereditary Genius*. (2nd Edition) London: Macmillan.

Gill, M. and Richards, T. (1998) Meeting the challenge of genetic advance. *British Medical Journal* 316: 570.

Hall, S., Bobrow, M. and Marteau T. (2000) Psychological consequences for parents of false negative results on prenatal screening for Down's syndrome: retrospective interview study. *British Medical Journal* 320: 407–412.

Holtzman, N. A. and Shapiro, D. (1998) The new genetics: genetic testing and public policy. *British Medical Journal* 316: 852–856.

Kitcher, P. (1997) *The lives to come: the genetic revolution and human possibilities*. Harmondsworth: Penguin Books.

Marteau, T. and Richards, M. (eds) (1996) *The troubled helix: social and psychological implications of the new human genetics*. Cambridge: Cambridge University Press.

Marteau, T. and Croyle, R.T. (1998) The new genetics: psychological responses to genetic testing. *British Medical Journal* 316: 693–696.

Mehlman, M.J. and Botkin, J.R. (1998) *Access to the genome: the challenge to equality*. Washington DC: Georgetown University Press.

Rioux, M. (1996) Reproductive technology: a rights issue. *Entourage* Summer 1996: 5–7.

Roeher Institute (1998) *Genomes and Justice – reflection on a holistic approach to Genetic Research, Technology and Disability*. Toronto: The Roeher Institute in co-operation with Inclusion International.

Shakespeare, T. (1997) Yallery Brown – a review of P. Kitcher (1997) The lives to come: the genetic revolution and human possibilities. *Disability and Society* 12: 485–487.

Snijders, R.J., Noble, P., Sebire, N., Souka, A. and Nicolaides, K.H. (1998) UK multicentre project on assessment of risk of trisomy 21 by maternal age and fetal nuchal-translucency thickness at 10–14 weeks of gestation. *Lancet* 352: 343–6.

Wald, N., Watt, H.C. and Hackshaw, A.K. (1999) Integrated screening for Down's syndrome on the basis of test performed during the first and second trimesters. *New England Journal of Medicine* 341: 521–522.

Wald, N., Huttly, W.J. and Hennessy, C.F. (1999) Down's syndrome screening in the UK in 1998. *Lancet* 354: 1264.

Weatherall, D. J. (1991), *The New Genetics and Clinical Practice*. Oxford: Oxford University Press

6. Some unanswered questions

Priscilla Alderson

Prenatal screening raises many questions. This chapter is about questions which have few answers, or which are hardly ever asked. I hope that the chapter is clear enough to be useful to a wide range of people. It was written during an early stage of the research project.

Why do we have prenatal screening?
Prenatal screening costs a lot of money. Unlike maternal screening, screening the foetus does not save lives or treat illness. Could we be doing better things with this money? Yet instead of asking *why* do we have prenatal screening, people usually talk about *how* can we do it better. Some important research looks at how anxious women become when they are screened (Marteau, 1989; Green and Statham, 1996). This work raises such questions as: 'If screening makes some people so anxious, is it worth doing?' Or at least it asks, 'How can we help people to be less anxious?' The work is fairly unusual, in raising critical questions about screening. Yet in an odd way, it implies that of course we must have screening *because* women are very anxious. There must, therefore, be a very serious danger which they are anxious about and which screening is meant to rescue them from. It is assumed we need to have screening to help people to cope with the dangers they are so anxious about. Before looking at the reasons for anxiety, the next question looks at what anxiety means.

What is anxiety?
The anxiety is hardly ever explained. It is called 'distress', 'clinical anxiety' or 'need for emotional support'. Doctors and nurses tend to see anxiety as a disease that they ought to treat, with reassurance, or support, or by removing the problem. Medicine, psychology, law and ethics all tend to split thinking from feeling, and to see feelings like anxiety as purely feeling. We talk about 'feeling anxious' but not about

'thinking anxious'. Yet no one can think without feeling or feel without thinking. Anxiety is partly thinking. You cannot simply 'be anxious'; you can only be anxious about something. If anxiety is seen as a vague feeling, an uncomfortable state, then if someone is worried, you might try to help them by cheering them up. So one aim of the screening staff is to say: "Your baby is all right, you don't need to worry." Another aim is to try to get rid of uncomfortable feelings. So if the staff say, "Your baby is not all right," they add, "So would you rather not have it?" – and then you can feel all right again.

Anxiety, which was often started by the screening in the first place, becomes the main problem. Suppose a test shows that the baby has Down's syndrome. Then screening staff say, "If you are worried, then we can get rid of your anxiety by getting rid of the foetus, of both the problems hidden inside you. But if you are not worried about having the baby, that is all right, we don't need to do anything". (Not doing anything means going through pregnancy and birth and bringing up the child.)

What are screened women anxious about?
Some women worry that they might have a late abortion. What would it be like? Some worry that they cannot understand all the medical details, or that they will not be able to make the 'right decision', or that they might have rows with their family about what they ought to do. Many women are horrified about having to decide whether to get rid of a baby they want to have – the most serious life-or-death decision they are ever likely to have to make.

I think there are two main reasons for these worries. One is that women fear that having a child with learning difficulties will mean endless hard work, sadness and no fun. It will be a burden for the whole family. The other (and I am guessing here) is so awful that hardly anyone talks about it, but (I think) it is fear of carrying and giving birth to a monster. A baby too unlike you to feel like your own child. An 'alien' that you will never be able to talk and laugh with. Someone who looks so different that other people will point and stare; not like the pretty babies in Mothercare books.

One reason for thinking that screening staff as well as many pregnant women are scared of 'monster myths' is the changing number of babies born with cleft lip or with talipes. Cleft lip involves a gap in the skin between the mouth and nose. After some operations this can hardly be noticed. With talipes, one or both feet are turned in. This too can be treated with surgery if it is severe enough, and it does not look ugly despite the awful name 'clubfoot'. Yet many fewer babies (per total births) are now born in the UK with these minor problems. Between 1982/3 and 1992, the birth rate figures for babies born with a cleft lip fell from 820 to 464 (that is they nearly halved in numbers) and the number of babies born with talipes fell from 2041 to 747 – that is roughly a third of the figures ten years earlier (Department of Health, 1994).

Why were so many fewer such babies born? Might it be that screening staff suggest considering abortion when they see these conditions on the scanning screen? But these conditions need not involve any serious difficulties except ignorant fear about them. So how much 'non-directive prenatal counselling' is based on incorrect views about disability, on fantasies rather than facts?

Why is there this fear about 'aliens'?
It is easier to be afraid of someone you have never met. Armies fight wars with people they do not know and can therefore see as very different and dangerous. The foetus is unseen. Meeting a new born baby, seeing and holding her, is quite unlike seeing a scan of a foetus with dark holes among the wriggling lines. When many disabled children go to special schools and grow up to be unemployed adults, most other people do not know disabled people, or have the chance to live and learn with them as friends. Doctors add to the fear of the unknown, the 'alien' and 'monster' myths when they casually talk of 'serious risk', 'fear', 'suffering', 'danger of handicap', 'abnormal', 'faulty', 'negative genes' and 'even worse problems'. . .

Medical textbooks and research about prenatal screening can increase ignorance and prejudice. One survey asked screening professionals if they agreed with abortion for certain conditions (Drake, Reid and Marteau, 1996). It explained that a child with spina bifida 'will be unable to walk' (many can, and others can perfectly easily use wheel chairs), and that cystic fibrosis involves 'an early death'. Many people with cystic fibrosis live into their thirties and now their forties. How early is an early death? People with Down's syndrome, the survey said, 'could communicate but are unable to live alone'. But quite a few people with Down's syndrome live on their own. And is *anyone* really able to 'live alone'? We all depend on one another.

Most people, including doctors, nurses and other screening staff, know very little about disabilities unless they happen to know a disabled person well. Medical books tend to give out-of-date information about learning difficulties, based on people who lived for years in long-stay institutions (the old 'mental handicap' hospitals). The books confuse the effects of a lonely, very boring, life with the effects of having a learning difficulty. They hardly ever report how some people with Down's syndrome now take GCSE exams, are employed, or travel across the world to take part in the paralympics.

Screening tests cannot tell how severe a condition might be or might become, and can say nothing about the kind of future life the person might live, or about changes in society. So prenatal screening tests can be as vague as reading tea leaves. The fear about 'aliens' grows when disabled people are treated as if they are separate and different; it disappears when disabled people are treated as ordinary members of society.

How could pregnant women get better information?
One idea is that pregnant women might visit a family with a child who has the same condition that their foetus has. Yet this falsely separates the condition from all other aspects of the life of the child and the whole family. Imagine that red hair is thought to be a big problem and a woman expecting a baby due to have red hair visits a family with a small boy with red hair. Suppose he has just kicked his football through the kitchen window and the woman arrives in the middle of a row about this. The boy's parents might try to hide their anger, or say that yes, their son demands a lot of hard work and patience, but maybe it is worth it – on the whole – and there are some good times.

How can any parents sum up their feelings about their child and 'advise' when they know that every family is so different? Something that is a dreadful crisis in one household, is a joke in another, or hardly noticed in a third. The idea of needing to visit to 'find out how a family manages to live with a condition' falsely emphasises doubt or dread about the condition, and suggests that it can be separated from the person and family concerned and generalised to another individual and their family.

Many disabled people argue that people generally will only become well informed about disability when they live alongside disabled people in all aspects of daily life. They will then know them as very varied individuals with a range of 'abilities' like the rest of the population. Prenatal screening programmes, however, work against inclusion policies because their purpose is to offer the 'choice' to expectant parents to exclude and reject an affected foetus. The programmes are built on negative assumptions about disability which make it impossible for the staff involved to be 'non-directive'.

What kinds of lives do people with inherited conditions actually live?
Life-style depends much more on money and policies than on genes. If you cannot walk, you can still have a busy social life if you have good transport. By 2002, all new taxis in Bristol will have to be able to take wheelchair users. Things are changing quickly. Many more children with learning difficulties go to mainstream schools, and show how capable they can be. Yet there is much more publicity about disabled people's limits than about their achievements. And even when successes are published, these are usually in a 'triumph over tragedy' format (Oliver, 1990) which implies that it is hard and unusual to succeed if you are disabled. 'Isn't it amazing that Tim has learning difficulties but he can win a gold medal!' We need much more research and publicity about the many positive sides of disabled people's lives.

How can research provide more information about life with learning difficulties?
Most research traditionally has concentrated on the 'difficulties'. Doctors and psychologists measure physical and mental 'problems'. They interview parents and concentrate on their worries. Societies like Mencap, Scope, and ones for autism or fragile X syndrome, as their newsletters show, sponsor and report research that also tends to

concentrate on problems and 'special needs'. They emphasise the inherited or 'disabling' condition as the central aspect of life, and work to raise funds for research to cure or relieve the condition. Many of the societies belong to the Genetic Interest Group that, as its name shows, sees genes and biology as the key factors.

Another perspective is to see social conditions like transport, school, income and work as having more important effects than genetic ones. Some families join social or sports groups rather than disability groups. Many say they do not see their child as different or disabled or as having special needs (Alderson and Goodey, 1998). Although professionals sometimes describe this as 'denial', it can be seen as the opposite, as acceptance and affirmation of all the ordinary aspects of life which their child can enjoy. Very few researchers interview people who themselves have inherited conditions, although their views may differ from those of their parents who are often assumed to speak for them.

The questions in our research

The European Commission sponsored a project in Finland, England, Greece and Holland on 'Prenatal Screening: Past, Present and Future, 1996–1999'. We asked doctors, nurses, experts, pregnant women and the general public for their views. As the most multiracial society involved, England also had a 'family survey'. We interviewed 40 people aged between 16 and 35, ten in each group of people who had sickle cell, thalassaemia or cystic fibrosis and five each who had Down's syndrome or spina bifida.

Prenatal screening is based on the view that the value and quality of life of people with these conditions may not be worthwhile. What did the people concerned think? The interviews looked at their views about the value and quality of their own life. What did they enjoy and find difficult? What were their aims and hopes? Were there any aspects of their life or society they would like to change? What did they feel about being or becoming partners or parents themselves? What were their views about screening and prenatal decisions? If they met someone who was expecting a baby with their condition, like Down's syndrome, what might they say to her?

It was recognised that some of these questions could be upsetting and painful. Should we ask them? If we did not, ignorance about the views of the most affected people would continue. The silence would imply that they could not cope with the questions, or even that they did not have any answers of their own. If someone gets upset, at least this will mean that they understand, and if so this could mean that they would like to talk even if it was upsetting. Nearly everyone in the study said that they felt all right talking about these questions; some said they welcomed the chance to do so. The exceptions were two men with Down's syndrome who had been talking eagerly about their work as actors. They suddenly became very sad. Words could not express their sadness about prenatal screening. Other people expressed acceptance; a few were angry.

How was this research unusual?

- Most research with people with learning difficulties sees them as 'patients' or 'dependent' in some way. This research saw them as people in their own right who contribute to society, and was about their views about their life.

- We aimed to work with them as partners, only tape recording if they agreed, and only talking about topics they were happy to talk about.

A lot is known about doctors' and nurses' views and quite a lot about parents', but very little about the views of the young people themselves.

- Interviews with young people with spina bifida 25 years ago found that many were very unhappy (for example, 85% in one study experienced depression, while 25% of the girls involved had had suicidal ideas, Dorner, 1976). But these studies tended not to take account of how their lives were made harder by the educational, social and medical policies of the time. Looking at the research today we can see the adverse impact on the young people's lives of medical policies then (eg spells in hospital at an early age at a time when visiting times were very restricted, Fulthorpe, 1974, Douglas, 1975), and educational policies too (young people at residential schools – ie away from their families – had much more negative feelings about school than their peers with spina bifida who went to ordinary or special day schools (Dorner, 1976). Children with similar medical conditions or impairments living at different times will have different life experiences as a result of the social policies, supports and attitudes prevalent in society.

- Emphasis on genes and the 'blue-print for life' tends to stereotype disabled groups and emphasise potential problems and costs. Our research aimed to redress the balance, by showing the great variety of their lives and the happy aspects of them as well.

- Talk about choice in prenatal screening respects the rights of future parents and of 'able' people. But if choice is to be informed, far more needs to be known about life with an inherited or potentially 'disabling' condition and the views of the people most directly concerned. For example, one woman with Down's syndrome talked about attempts to exclude her from school. The interviewer said, "So you had a row about it?" She answered, "No, not a row, a fight, a fight for my rights".

- Professionals need to know more about the views of the people they want to help, if they are to plan useful health and screening services. Our research was intended to help everyone to be able to make more informed prenatal decisions (Alderson, 1999; Goodey et al, 1999).

References

Alderson, P. (1999) The good life? *Bulletin of Medical Ethics* 147: 15–16.

Alderson, P. and Goodey, C. (1998) *Enabling education: experiences in special and ordinary schools.* London: Tufnell Press.

Department of Health (1994) *Health and personal social services statistics for England 1994 edition* Table 4.3: 24. London: HMSO.

Dorner, S. (1976) Adolescents with spina bifida: how they see their situation. *Archives of Disease in Childhood* 51, 6: 439–444.

Douglas, J.W.B. (1975) Early hospital admissions and later disturbances of behaviour and learning. *Developmental Medicine and Child Neurology* 17, 4: 456–480.

Drake, H., Reid, M. and Marteau T. (1996) Attitudes towards termination for fetal abnormality: comparisons in three European countries. *Clinical Genetics* 49, 3: 134–140.

Fulthorpe, D. (1974) Spina bifida: some psychological aspects. *Special Education* 1, 4: 17–20.

Goodey, C., Alderson, P. and Appleby, J. (1999) The ethical implications of ante natal screening for Down's syndrome. *Bulletin of Medical Ethics* 147: 7–13.

Green, J. and Statham, H. (1996) Psychological aspects of prenatal screening and diagnosis. In T. Marteau and M. Richards (eds) *The troubled helix: social and psychological implications of the new human genetics*. Cambridge: Cambridge University Press.

Marteau, T. (1989) Psychological costs of screening. *British Medical Journal* 299: 527.

Oliver, M. (1990) *The politics of disablement*. Basingstoke: Macmillan.

7. 'Three generations of imbeciles are enough':
eugenics, the new genetics and people with learning difficulties

Agnes Fletcher

Introduction

The Human Genome Project – the Holy Grail of health and the biggest scientific enterprise of the century – is providing fascinating information about the way the human body functions and develops. It also brings new threats to the lives and well-being of already disadvantaged individuals, whose genes and characteristics may soon be exploited by others for profit.

I would like to provide a disability equality perspective on the subject of genetics and people with learning difficulties. I will look in turn at the history of genetics and disability; at current practice – focusing particularly on genetic screening during pregnancy; and provide some suggestions to uphold the human rights of people with learning difficulties in relation to genetics.

Eugenics

Disabled people are in an ideal position to warn the rest of society about how the science of genetics may be used for evil ends. Genetics has an unhappy history, to put it mildly, and for those of us with genetic impairments, this is part of our history. Many disabled people are anxious that the mass sterilisation and murder that occurred in the name of genetics in the early part of this century, which led to the extermination of people on the basis of other traits deemed hereditary, were not a Nazi anomaly but an extreme instance of a deep-seated hostility towards, and fear of, impairments.

It certainly is not my intention to insult the many scientists engaged in valuable research or to suggest that we are on the brink of state atrocities. However, geneticists look at the intimate details of our family histories to throw light on the present and to prevent or reduce future dangers. Looking at our collective history as disabled people may help to avoid further abuses of the science of genetics.

This is familiar territory but worth repeating. In 1930s Germany, there were around 400,000 compulsory sterilisations of disabled people. A list of genetic and psychiatric conditions was drawn up for which killing was permitted. A system of genetic health courts was established. Each tribunal had a lawyer, a medical officer and a doctor with specialist training in 'racial hygiene'. Thousands of disabled people were killed. These policies, and the sophisticated methods of mass killing developed later, destroyed millions of members of other groups seen as undesirable to German society.

In other parts of Europe and in America, as recent newspaper reports have revealed, mass sterilisation programmes for eugenic purposes continued until very recently, focused particularly on 'the feeble-minded'. The landmark US Supreme Court case of 1927 upheld the right to forcibly sterilise Carrie Buck, supposed to be 'feeble-minded'. The judge, reflecting in his judgement that the nation's 'best' citizens might be called upon to give up their lives in war, said of sterilising the feeble-minded or insane:

> *It would be strange if we could not call upon those who already sap the strength of the state for these lesser sacrifices . . . It is better for all the world if, instead of waiting to execute degenerate offspring for crime, or to let them starve for their imbecility, society can prevent those who are manifestly unfit from continuing their kind . . . Three generations of imbeciles are enough.*

David, Smith and Nelson, 1989

More recently, in 1994, China introduced its own eugenics Maternal and Infant Health Care law to reduce the number of 'inferior births'. Among other provisions, this allows the state to prevent people with disabilities from marrying or having children.

Genetics or eugenics?

Choices regulating reproduction in the United Kingdom are mostly implemented by individual women and men, rather than as the consequence of state intervention. Nevertheless, as I shall stress later, there are considerable pressures on prospective parents which undermine the exercise of free choice, and this is particularly the case for people with learning difficulties and other disabled people.

The Nuffield Council on Bioethics has acknowledged, in its 1993 report *Genetic Screening: Ethical Issues*, that the 'potential of eugenic misuse of genetic testing will increase' as genetics develops. Indeed, research and experience clearly reveal a tendency to assume the desirability of preventing the birth of foetuses with certain conditions (see below and Alderson, chapter 6, this volume) and thus attribute, by implication, a negative value to people living with those conditions.

Prenatal screening

Tests during pregnancy are offered to the majority of women in this country. Until the late 1980s, the main tests available were designed to detect spina bifida and Down's syndrome. Now, up to one hundred conditions are detectable in the womb (including bowel cancer, cystic fibrosis and muscular dystrophy). There are huge pressures on all parents to test and, following a 'bad' result, to terminate. Over 90% of those who know that their foetus has Down's syndrome terminate the pregnancy. Live births of infants with spina bifida have dropped rapidly in recent years – possibly as a result of folic acid supplements; almost certainly as a result of increased effectiveness of prenatal diagnosis and subsequent termination (see Alderson, chapter 6 this volume). Some of the pressures on parents come from directiveness or bias during the information-giving and counselling process.

A survey by the National Childbirth Trust (NCT) on the stress of tests in pregnancy found that the right of parents to choose not to have prenatal screening was undermined by some health professionals' assumption that screening, and termination of pregnancy in the case of impairment, was always the best option (Dodds, 1997). The NCT's Policy Research Officer, Rosemary Dodds, commented:

The technology for antenatal screening is outstripping the counselling available. Some of the parents we heard from had received crass treatment. We need multi-disciplinary training for all those health professionals involved, so that they provide clear, accurate information to parents in a sensitive way.

Fletcher, 1997

In addition there are cultural, financial and commercial pressures at play, affecting prospective parents and disabled people generally.

Cultural pressures affecting choice
Overwhelmingly, the media represent testing and termination on the grounds of impairment as an agonising problem but an inevitable choice. The birth of a disabled child is seen as nothing other than a tragedy for the family and for that child, as these headlines from recent British newspapers demonstrate:

A cruel inheritance   To screen or not to screen

'Bad genes' abortion call   The gene detective

There's something wrong with your baby

Dilemma of the faulty genes   My son should have been aborted

The agony of making a choice

The hardest choice of all   The baby dilemma that won't go away

The choice no mother ever wants to make

There are a huge number of magazine and newspaper articles about this 'agonising' choice. While the views of those who choose to maintain a pregnancy once impairment is diagnosed are sometimes represented, overwhelmingly the attitude of most commentators is that impairment is a tragedy to be avoided at all costs. The decision to terminate is usually represented as in the interests of the child: the life of a person with a genetic condition is one of such suffering that it is better that they are not born. So, while bringing a disabled child into the world remains a 'choice', it becomes a selfish action causing suffering.

Financial pressures

As well as sparing the supposed suffering of the prospective child, prenatal tests are also justified by their cost-effectiveness. The *British Medical Journal* reported some years ago that, while screening costs up to £38,000 to 'avoid the birth of a Down's syndrome child', this could be balanced against the estimated lifetime costs of £120,000 (Wald et al, 1992; see also Sheldon et al, 1991). Access to tests may be linked to willingness to terminate in the case of impairment. Where some parents might like the chance to prepare for the birth of a baby with an impairment, this opportunity may be denied as testing would then cease to be 'cost-effective'.

In addition to the economic imperative behind the new technology, the inadequacy of economic and social support for parents of disabled children has been proved again and again (Beresford, 1995; Dobson and Middleton, 1998; Joseph Rowntree Foundation, 1999). These pressures, together with the lack of support and opportunities for disabled adults to participate fully in society, mean that the 'choice' to parent a disabled child is in effect denied, particularly if the parent is also disabled.

Technological pressures

From what I can gather, practice within health authorities in relation to genetic screening is being driven by the technology and resources available, not by any consistent national policy informed by public debate about the ethical and social implications of these fast-changing developments. This is far from ideal. While there are clearly a great many good genetic counsellors, the variation in service provision nationwide and the fact that practice is being driven by technology, not policy, is dangerous.

Commercial pressures

The commercialisation of conception, with press speculation of bespoke embryos with the 'right' characteristics available in the future at a price, signals an increasing interest in the control of 'product quality'.

As far as genetics research is concerned, many researchers are engaged in valuable, ethical research, designed to help understand and overcome disease, often funded by biotechnology companies. However, much of the research is leading to tests rather than treatments, which are extremely lucrative, especially if patented. The existence of a test creates demand for its widespread availability, even when the condition tested for is extremely rare.

To give an example, as far as treatment is concerned, shortness as a perceived impairment has meant the marketability of human growth hormone, made by genetic engineering and developed originally for those with growth hormone deficiency. Since the mid-1980s, biotechnology companies have persuaded doctors to prescribe it to children in the shortest 3% of the population – whether or not they have a growth hormone deficiency. The availability of the treatment has led to thousands of parents, worried at the prospect of their children being bullied or discriminated against, pumping hormones into them, thus lining the pockets of the biotechnology companies.

The myth of objectivity

'Give them the facts and let them choose'. It is a mantra that totally ignores social context, assumes that there is a neat selection of facts that are relevant and expects that information can be delivered in a way that is not heavily laden with the values of the messenger and is understood by everyone in the same way. I am consciously choosing the facts that I assemble to back up my argument. That choice is driven by my perspective on this subject, as a person with an inheritable impairment. I acknowledge that there are unconscious factors, relating to my upbringing and my culture which, while impossible to enumerate, undoubtedly affect my choice and presentation of these facts. Without proper debate about the nature of impairment and disability in society, and without the voices and experiences of disabled people being readily available during the counselling process, we are further from the ideal of objectivity than we need be.

Extra pressures on people with learning difficulties

While any prospective parent may experience the pressures outlined above, the situation for people with learning difficulties who may wish to become parents is particularly difficult. For example, they are likely to experience enormous problems trying to exercise their rights in the area of relationships, sex and reproduction. Pregnancy for people with learning difficulties is almost always viewed as a disaster – something that should have been prevented. This applies to an even greater extent should tests reveal that the foetus is 'impaired' and the woman or couple want to keep the child. People with learning difficulties also have particular problems getting easy-to-understand information and non-directive counselling. Most public information remains inaccessible to them and if parenting a disabled child is generally discouraged via prenatal testing even for non-disabled parents, how much harder is it for prospective parents with learning difficulties to continue a pregnancy when a disabling condition has been diagnosed.

Conclusion

So how would I summarise the potential benefits of genetic screening and research and the potential disadvantages involved? And what can we do to safeguard the rights and interests of people with learning difficulties in this area?

Potential benefits of genetic screening and research

- Prevention of impairments with genetic and environmental triggers.

- Potential future reduction in the incidence of impairment by methods other than selective termination – such as gene manipulation, gene therapy and other treatments.

- Targeting of resources and prevention strategies.

- Reassurance from a diagnosis brings comfort to many parents and helps them and others involved in the care of young children to cope with challenging behaviour and to discover the best methods of supporting and educating such children. Having a diagnosis can overcome accusations of bad parenting.

Disadvantages of genetic testing and screening

- Genetic discrimination – for example, in education, employment or insurance. This is already happening (see Rioux, chapter 9 this volume). In terms of social policy more generally, the American book *The bell curve* on intelligence argued that resources put into improving the education of disadvantaged groups are wasted because these people are genetically destined to be low achievers (Herrnstein and Murray, 1994). While such books represent an extreme, they indicate that such ideas in a more diluted form may have an influence.

- Genetic determinism – the belief that it is genes that affect individuals' health status (with an associated loss of motivation for individuals and society to try to improve health through lifestyle, diet, not smoking and other choices).

- Geneticisation of differences – everything from height and weight, to personality and intelligence – may be (inaccurately) perceived as wholly genetically determined and medicalised as a result. For example, to be much shorter than average means you are ill (literally sub-standard), in need of (expensive) tests and treatment, and thus vulnerable to commercial exploitation (see Ward, chapter 1 this volume).

- Those who might prove good parents in many ways are already deciding against parenting purely on the basis of their genetic status.

- Effects on individual identity and family life – feeling 'genetically tainted'; an inadequate partner; someone who should not reproduce.

- Stigmatisation – of those who knowingly pass on 'bad genes'; possibly even 'punishment', such as withdrawal of benefits; and labelling (people's genetic condition becomes their label).

- Increased anxiety about oneself and one's potential children, particularly during pregnancy.

Safeguarding the rights and interests of people with learning difficulties

To safeguard the rights and interests of disabled people and people with learning difficulties in this area we need to act to ensure:

- Increased and continuing public debate – to match the pace of change and the scale of the 'Genetic Revolution' – including public information and debate about the direction in which research and screening/testing policies are moving.

- Nationally recognised standards and guidelines for health authorities on prenatal testing, screening and associated issues.

- Monitoring and regulation of research, which should incorporate the perspective of disabled people in this area.

- Support for the choices of people with learning difficulties in deciding to become parents, and afterwards in parenting.

- Promotion of accessible and, as far as possible, 'objective' information and counselling for people with learning difficulties and support throughout pregnancy.

- Involvement of disabled people (including people with learning difficulties) in genetic counselling.

- Public awareness of the fact that people can be good or bad parents, whether or not they have an impairment.

- Outlawing of discrimination against people on the grounds of their genes.

- A reduction in medical solutions based on social prejudice. For example, surgery for children with Down's syndrome has had recent media coverage. Some of this surgery may have a therapeutic benefit – for example, surgery on the tongue to stop dribbling and infections. But some of it seems to have no clinical basis (for example, surgery on the eyes) and is designed to overcome societal prejudices by altering the individual (in a sense locating the blame for that prejudice within the individual). Procedures which carry some risk, however small, which have no medical benefit should be left until children are older and better able to understand and consent to such a procedure.

- Disabled people should neither be coerced into, nor denied the opportunity of benefiting from, screening programmes.

There are undoubtedly benefits to genetic testing and genetic research but the dangers for disabled people are clear: an increased sense that our lives are not worth living and should be ended as soon as we are detected: more disability discrimination.

References

Beresford, B. (1995) *Expert opinions: a national survey of parents caring for a severely disabled child*. Bristol: Policy Press/*Community Care*.

David, J., Smith, K. and Nelson, R. (1989) *Against her will: the Carrie Buck story*. New Horizon Press.

Dobson, B. and Middleton, S. (1998) *Paying to care: the cost of childhood disability*. York: York Publishing Services.

Dodds, R. (1997) *The stress of tests in pregnancy. Summary of a National Childbirth Trust antenatal screening survey*. London: National Childbirth Trust.

Fletcher, A. (1997) It's not the baby's responsibility to be perfect. *Amazons* (Newsletter of British Council of Disabled People's Women's Group) June: 1, 4, 5.

Herrnstein, R.J. and Murray, C. (1994) *The bell curve: intelligence and class structure in American life*. New York: Free Press.

Joseph Rowntree Foundation (1999) Supporting disabled children and their families. *Foundations* N79. York: Joseph Rowntree Foundation.

Nuffield Council on Bioethics (1993) *Genetic screening: ethical issues*. London: Nuffield Council on Bioethics.

Sheldon, T.A. and Simpson, J (1991) Prenatal screening for Down's syndrome (letter). *British Medical Journal* 303: 55–6.

Wald, N.J., Kennard, A, Densem, J.W., Cuckle, H.S., Chard, T and Butler, L. (1992) Antenatal maternal serum screening for Down's syndrome: results of a demonstration project. *British Medical Journal* 305: 391–4.

8. Whose choice? Whose responsibility?

Ethical issues in prenatal diagnosis and learning disability

Ruth Chadwick

Introduction

The issues surrounding developments in human genome analysis, and the implications of discoveries of certain genetic conditions, are extremely controversial, partly because of fears born of historical precedents of the abuse of genetics. Prenatal diagnosis gives rise to ethical questions primarily because of its association with the possibility of termination of pregnancy, which remains a highly contested issue.

This chapter does not attempt to 'settle' the issues around termination. Rather, the questions to be addressed include the ethics of screening foetuses for learning disabilities, with the possibility of termination of foetuses found to be affected. From one point of view this constitutes unjustifiable discrimination against those with a learning disability; from another point of view it may be seen as facilitating choice for the parents. What is required is a set of criteria for judging what is acceptable and what is not acceptable. I shall *not* be discussing any scientific 'facts' about any genetic basis of learning disabilities. But the fact that any possible genetic basis is *not* clearly understood, does affect the ethical acceptability of undertaking genetic testing and screening and of drawing conclusions from the results.

Termination of pregnancies is a fact of life in our society. The Abortion Act of 1967, as amended by the Human Fertilisation and Embryology Act of 1990, defines the conditions under which the procurement of termination is not unlawful. These include a clause referring to disorders which are seriously handicapping (cf Morgan and Lee, 1991).

A termination will not be unlawful where:

> *. . . there is a substantial risk that if the child were born it would suffer from such physical or mental abnormalities as to be seriously handicapped.*

Abortion Act, 1967

Some conceptual clarifications are in order. 'Genetic testing' is carried out on an individual who, there is reason to believe, is at risk of a certain condition (for example, because of family history). 'Population (genetic) screening' is the process of establishing, over a given population or subset of a population, the frequency of occurrence of a gene or chromosome type, where there is no reason to believe that any particular individual has the genetic characteristic in question. The distinction is not entirely clear-cut, because there is disagreement as to whether certain subsets of populations constitute 'at risk' groups for testing (for example, because membership of the group, rather than individual history, constitutes a risk) or satisfy the requirements for screening (cf Chadwick et al, 1997). Whether testing or screening is at stake, the ethical issues overlap to a large extent but differ in certain ways – for example, public health goals are likely to be a determining factor in whether or nor it is considered worthwhile to put public resources into a screening programme.

What is the condition?
There is an influential view that, in order to justify the implementation of a screening programme, the condition sought has to be 'serious' (cf Nuffield Council on Bioethics, 1993). What counts as 'serious', however, is in dispute. It might be tempting to think in terms of conditions that are life-threatening or severely disabling. Where learning disabilities are concerned, however, the issue is particularly fraught. Not only is there a variety of conditions (genetic and chromosomal) potentially involved – from fragile X syndrome to Down's syndrome, for example – but also the extent to which they are disabling varies both objectively and subjectively. Objectively, the severity of manifestation of a genetic condition may vary widely; subjectively, the extent to which the disability handicaps an individual is likely also to differ. From one point

of view 'handicap' is constructed by society and should be resolved by society; from another point of view (not *necessarily* incompatible with this) it may still be felt by some to be important to attempt to alleviate the genetic basis of whatever it is that is deemed to be at the root of social handicap.

The very fact that a condition *is* deemed serious by some parts of the community may be perceived as potentially discriminatory by those who have a learning disability or represent people who do. Translating that perception into action, in the form of prenatal screening and possibly termination, may be seen as a violation of the rights of people with learning disabilities who are currently alive.

Much of the controversy surrounding the nature-nurture debate, eugenics and genetic screening, has concentrated on intelligence. This says something about the values of society. In the 1980s, Singapore tried a modern experiment of a eugenic sort when it appeared that highly educated and intelligent women were not marrying and producing children for the future benefit of Singapore society. Incentives were introduced for them to find partners and reproduce (Chan, 1992). Criticisms of such efforts have focused on the limited understanding of genetics underlying them and on the interference with freedom involved. In present day society, moreover, it is not necessarily intelligence that is likely to produce either a happy or successful life in a particular social context; physical prowess might be a better bet.

The point of this discussion is to show that notions of what count as 'seriously handicapping' and of what count as advantages, from a genetic point of view, are highly contested.

What can be done?
There is little point in undertaking any kind of screening programme unless some positive intervention will be forthcoming in the light of a positive result. But the idea of a 'positive' result is itself not clear. Would-be screeners have to deal with the possibility of both 'false negative' and 'false positive' results. What is desired is a test sufficiently specific to minimise false positives and sufficiently sensitive to minimise false negatives (Shickle and Chadwick, 1994).

In the case of some disorders with a genetic factor involved, there are forms of therapy that can ameliorate the condition. One of the most commonly cited examples of this is phenylketonuria (PKU) which can be treated by dietary therapy. In the case of other conditions, such as cystic fibrosis, the possibility of 'gene therapy' in the future is mooted. Discussions of the desirability of testing for fragile X syndrome, however, have focused on the lack of a cure, which is particularly important where the testing of children is concerned (Webb, 1994).

The Danish Council of Ethics has suggested there must be some 'scope for action' in order to justify screening (Danish Council of Ethics, 1993). This encompasses a range of possibilities wider than therapy, and can include termination and decision-making of various kinds. Where prenatal diagnosis for learning disabilities is concerned, the potential intervention may be limited to termination of pregnancy, rather than the possibility of amelioration of the situation *for the person that the foetus would become*. Hence, unless a case can be made out for the possibility of 'wrongful life' (the suggestion that an individual might be harmed and even wronged by being brought into existence, because his or her life would be of such poor quality), the scope for action is to the benefit of potential parents rather than those who actually have the condition. Genetic technology is often presented as producing benefits in terms of choice (based on relevant genetic information). But this choice may be to prevent a person from coming into being rather than to opt for some type of therapy.

The distinction between these different types of case is not entirely clear-cut – for example, some might argue that gene therapy may have identity-changing results; the person after therapy might be perceived as a different person from the person before therapy (Elliott, 1993). One might say that the original person has been killed and a new person brought into being. (Some might argue that this is different from procuring a termination since the actual death of the original person was not aimed at here.)

It is not the purpose of the present discussion to investigate the rights or wrongs of termination *per se*. But where the termination of disabled foetuses is the issue, it is readily understandable if people with learning difficulties currently alive feel that they are the object of discriminatory practices that actually amount to a desire for their elimination.

There are powerful logical arguments to the effect that this is not the case – that it is not *persons* with disabilities that are being treated differently, but foetuses. It is not unlawful under the Abortion Act 1967 (as amended by the Human Fertilisation and Embryology Act 1990) to terminate the life of a foetus which there is no reason to think is anything other than a paradigm of health, if certain conditions are satisfied. Perhaps some people currently alive who consider themselves healthy find this threatening; the evidence suggests most do not. Some disabled people and their allies, however, do find the testing and termination of foetuses with certain conditions threatening.

Here, it is not sufficient to argue that logically the dividing line is between foetuses and more developed forms of life, rather than between those with certain disabilities and those without. Both symbolism and practical steps are important. From a symbolic point of view, we may ask why it is necessary to have a separate clause in the abortion law referring to handicap (or indeed why access to termination on the grounds of a foetus being disabled is possible throughout pregnancy whereas termination on other grounds is not permitted after 24 weeks). Simple reference to the choice and/or welfare of the mother and her family might be preferable. Practically, an eye must be had to the social context in which decisions are made. If the social context is such that it is not feasible for would-be parents to give adequate care to offspring with certain conditions, then discrimination might indeed be a fact of life. The important point to note is that it does not follow from the very fact of prenatal screening and termination *itself* that discrimination is being carried out against persons with disabilities (though the differential time limits for termination of 'disabled' and 'non-disabled' foetuses could be seen to be discriminatory).

It is important to note that termination need not *necessarily* follow prenatal diagnosis. Despite arguments suggesting that people should not enter into prenatal diagnosis unless they are prepared to accept a termination in the light of a positive result (partly because of resource implications) prenatal diagnosis could, on the contrary, provide the opportunity for parents to prepare for the care of a child with a certain condition.

Autonomy and choice

Present-day clinical genetics presents itself, to a considerable extent, as being concerned with the provision of information, to allow individuals and couples to make informed choices, largely (but not exclusively) about reproduction. In the case of prenatal diagnosis of a foetus with a (learning) disability, the idea is that knowing this would provide the parents with the opportunity to decide, freely, whether to opt for a termination or to prepare for the upbringing of the child.

Whether or not genetic information promotes autonomous choice, however, is increasingly questioned, from at least three points of view. First, it is necessary to have regard to the context in which choices are made. A social environment hostile or indifferent to certain forms of disability does not facilitate genuine choice. Second, the amount of genetic information forthcoming (which may be relatively poorly understood) may turn out to be a burden to parents rather than a help (Danish Council of Ethics, 1993). Third, there is more than one possible interpretation of autonomy. Autonomy may not simply be a matter of having a great deal of information on the basis of which a decision should be taken. On the contrary, it may mean the right not to know certain genetic information (Husted, 1997).

What are the arguments for a right not to know? They may be divided into those that concern the value of knowledge in itself; those that concern the consequences for the individual; and those relating to the consequences for society.

Is genetic knowledge valuable in itself? In the absence of details about who has this knowledge it is difficult to give any sense to this question. Then the answer must surely depend on their position and priorities – in which case the answer to the question appears to be 'no'.

For the individual, the knowledge may be experienced as a beneficial release from uncertainty or as the onset of anxiety. In society, genetic knowledge may have consequences so far-reaching that it has been argued that research should not even be done into the genetic basis of certain features of human life (cf Shickle, 1997). Any genetic basis of intelligence may be one candidate for such exclusion, given the potential for educational and other forms of discrimination (which may possibly lead in turn to self-fulfilling prophecies) and deterministic thinking.

If autonomy is taken to mean that individuals should be free to define themselves rather than to be labelled or stigmatised, then providing information about the genetic basis of your intelligence or that of your foetus cannot necessarily be seen as autonomy-enhancing, just because it provides additional information to feed into decision-making. Hence the arguments for a right not to know; but these can also be challenged.

Arguments against a right not to know

Medical ethics has for a long time been concerned with the rights of patients and clients to have access to information, as a reaction to traditional paternalism on the part of health care professionals. The move to a right *not to know* is relatively new, but is itself challenged, not only in terms of the long-standing debates about autonomy and paternalism, but also in the light of newer discussions about autonomy and community. The communitarian turn in ethics (particularly relevant in genetics because the latter emphasises the relatedness of individuals who share the same genes) has opened the way to talk of solidarity and of responsible parenthood. The idea of responsible parenthood might be interpreted in terms of duties to make, if not certain sorts of reproductive decisions, at least decisions in the light of as much relevant information as possible, including genetic information (Royal College of Physicians, 1991). Solidarity with the group may imply the desirability of sharing genetic information (Berg, 1994).

If we are to talk in terms of solidarity and responsibility, however, we have to ask who has responsibility for whom, and who should show solidarity with whom. One sense of solidarity is grounded in the idea that individuals with 'special needs' should not be abandoned to their fate, but that society has a responsibility to provide sufficient welfare to support them by making appropriate services available. Without this commitment the logical arguments distinguishing between issues of screening and termination on the one hand, and of discrimination on the other, sound rather hollow.

Conclusion

The future possibilities regarding the practical implications of discoveries concerning the genetic basis of learning disabilities can only be a matter of speculation. It may be that they might lead to ways of improving cognitive abilities (Vines, 1996).

At present, however, the issues under discussion apply mainly to parents having their children or foetuses tested. In the former case, it is suggested that it may provide parental comfort to know the cause of their child's difficulties; in the latter, it raises the issue of termination. The issues may be constructed in terms of the competing values of parental choice, the welfare of the future child and the implications for people in society with these disabilities. To argue for a right to know, on the grounds of autonomy and choice, is insufficient; claims of a right not to know because of the potential burdens of genetic information without compensating benefits are increasingly heard, but are challenged by notions of responsibility, especially responsible parenthood. The question that must be asked, however, is who has responsibility to whom. A communitarian ethics cannot stop at the responsibilities of individuals to society but must include a mutuality of responsibility, which will include provision of support for those with 'special needs'. Otherwise there can be no genuine choice, and support will be given to the argument that genetic screening and testing are in effect, if not in intention, discriminatory.

References

Berg, K. (1994) The need for laws, rules and good practices to secure optimal disease control. In *Ethics and human genetics* 122–134. Strasbourg: Council of Europe.

Chadwick, R., Levitt, M. and Shickle, D. (eds) (1997) *The right to know and the right not to know*. Aldershot: Avebury.

Chan, C.K. (1992) Eugenics on the rise: a report from Singapore. In R. F. Chadwick *Ethics, reproduction and genetic control* 2nd edition 164–71. London: Routledge.

Danish Council of Ethics (1993) *Ethics and the mapping of the human genome.* Copenhagen: Danish Council of Ethics.

Elliott, R. (1993) Identity and the ethics of gene therapy. *Bioethics* 7: 27–40

Husted, J. (1997) Autonomy and a right not to know. In R. Chadwick, M.A. Levitt and D. Shickle (eds) *The right to know and the right not to know.* Aldershot: Avebury.

Morgan, D. and Lee, R.G. (1991) *Blackstone's guide to the Human Fertilisation and Embryology Act 1990.* London: Blackstone Press.

Nuffield Council on Bioethics (1993) *Genetic screening: ethical issues.* London: Nuffield Council on Bioethics.

Royal College of Physicians (1991) *Ethical issues in clinical genetics.* London: Royal College of Physicians.

Shickle, D. (1997) Do 'all men desire to know'? A right of society to choose not to know about the genetics of personality traits. In R. Chadwick, M.A. Levitt and D. Shickle (eds) *The right to know and the right not to know.* Aldershot: Avebury.

Shickle, D. and Chadwick, R. (1994) The ethics of screening: is 'screening-itis' an incurable disease? *Journal of Medical Ethics* 20: 12–18.

Vines, G. (1996) The search for the clever stuff. *Guardian* 1 February.

Webb, J. (1994) A fragile case for screening? *New Scientist* 25 December 1993/1 January 1994, 10–11.

9. The many interests in genetic knowledge:

an international perspective on prenatal screening and the use of genetic information in relation to people with learning difficulties

Marcia Rioux

Prenatal screening and genetic information are usually thought of as medical issues. While prenatal screening may take place in a hospital or in a clinic and while genetic counselling may be attached to medical professionals, the real issues that emerge from these practices are to be found elsewhere.

What are the issues then? Some of the questions raised by lay people in different countries about prenatal screening and genetic information include:

- What is the Human Genome Project?

- How much money is involved in this kind of technology?

- How important is prenatal screening and the use of genetic information in making the world a better place?

- Do prenatal screening and genetic information relieve suffering?

- Would someone want to be born with an intellectual disability? Is it better not to be born at all than to be born with a disability?

- Are people really determined by their genes?

- Can a person who understands genes really predict what another person's life will be like?

- Are there some people who are asking questions about the effects of genetic screening and genetic information on different groups of people?

- What does choice mean in an 'ablist' world (that is, a world which privileges non-disabled people)?

These are just some of the questions that are asked in different ways in a variety of contexts. They raise the issue of what is meant by 'an international perspective' in this field. In trying to frame an international perspective, I started by thinking about people's different cultural and national experiences but I realised that I was hearing similar questions in different countries – questions that seemed to cut across cultural lines and were extraneous to national experiences. The questions seem to be driven much more by the type of vested interests groups have than by nationalities. And so I will step back and reflect on the different parties and perspectives that have arisen in this field and the way the issues have been framed by them.

The identifiable interests that seem to predominate and that have publicly staked claims in the debates and discussions include genomics, law, commerce, genetic counselling, policy design and development, bioethics, rights advocacy and the social sciences.

Each of these frame the scientific, theoretical and political issues in a somewhat different manner and each sees itself as having some prior and over-riding moral claim to leadership or supremacy in the field. Some raise procedural questions and issues and some raise substantive issues and questions; they also differ with respect to the way in which they professionalise the field of genetics. Some are more influential in influencing the discourse and the direction of the field. An exploration of these perspectives, while not exhaustive, provides a flavour of the discussions that are taking place. They also bring to light the reasons why the public discussion is a difficult one and make it clear that perspectives, issues and priorities are not shared.

The perspective of the science of genes
The Human Genome Project (HUGO) is history's largest biological research collaboration. Launched in 1990 and sponsored by the US Department of Energy (DOE), the National Institutes of Health and the Wellcome Trust, its goal is to map each of the approximately 30,000 human genes to their location on the human chromosomes and to

sequence the order of the three billion nucleotide base pairs that make up the human DNA. The United States government has committed $3 billion to the project over a 15 year period. Many other countries are involved in the genome project, funded through their own governments and private biotechnological companies. France, the UK, Japan, Australia, Denmark, Italy, Russia, Germany and Canada are involved in the research, to name just a few countries.

Knowledge of the genetic code and an understanding of its orderly translation are generally regarded by scientists as the fundamental keys to human biological structure and function. While the weight given to this information in terms of understanding what makes us human is not unanimous among scientists, there is no doubt that the knowledge will have profound effects on human health and disease and on the perception of human origin and place in the natural world. The Human Genome Project is termed by many as a 'major new science' and the findings as the 'most significant intellectual discovery in humanity's scientific evolution' (Gert, 1966).

Prenatal screening and testing are two of the many new reproductive technologies and information sources that are generated from this work. The range of interventions include: abortion, contraception, amniocentesis, cloning, *in vitro* fertilisation, alternative insemination by spouse or donor, sperm banks, storage of frozen sperm, and genetic engineering. Presented as a triumph of modern science, advocates of the new reproductive technology make claims that this technology opens up the range of reproductive choices available to parents and will lead to a decrease of disability and disease in society.

The purpose of genomic research is to understand the genetic basis of human physical characteristics. Understanding the psychological and behavioural aspects of our being is also part of this research although this is infinitely more complex because of the interplay with environmental factors.

For some, genomics is a purely scientific enterprise, the consequences of which can be left to others. This view of the scientific inquiry of genetics is what Margaret Somerville calls '. . . a profoundly biological view of human identity, a gene machine approach' (Somerville, 1996) in which advancing scientific knowledge about genes and genetic technology is self-justifying.

Thus, for example, when a scientist who had announced in the late 1990s that he had found the first marker for intelligence (which he claimed would bring great benefit to neuroscience and society) was asked about the ethics of his research, he replied that he was just doing basic science and was not concerned with the ethics of it.

Ian Wilmut, the scientist who cloned Dolly the sheep, proposed that rather than use human clones as material for transplants, cloned pigs could provide organs that would be readily transplantable to humans. The question he posed was:

> How do you come up with a source of organs for the roughly 160,000 people a year in the developed world who die before an organ becomes available for transplant?

> *Toronto Star*, March 13, 1997

Other scientists are said to been involved in the development of headless frogs which they maintain could produce human organ-bearing torsos – a claim called 'repugnant and nonsensical' by Wilmut (ibid). Such are the debates of gene scientists.

Wilmut reflects the line of thinking of many scientists of genetics, however, in claiming that while human cloning (and no doubt some other forms of genetic engineering) is 'morally wrong' and should be 'legally prohibited', research into cloning should be allowed to continue.

> My view of this question is we should be very ambitious in our research, but then be very cautious in the way we use new knowledge.

> *Toronto Star*, March 13, 1997

This suggests that only those who *apply* the research should be carefully controlled and that scientific research itself should be given free rein.

The perspective of commercial and economic interests

There are dozens of companies that have been set up in the past few years whose singular goal is to discover and commercialise DNA sequences that make up human genes. With names like Human Genome Sciences, Myriad Genetics, Gen Vec and Genomyx, these corporations have investments from such pharmaceutical giants as SmithKline Beecham and Hoffman-LaRoche. It is estimated that the established pharmaceutical corporations' investment in genome research companies is over one billion dollars (Cohen, 1997). Erramouspe notes:

> *SmithKline Beecham committed $125 million (US) last year (1995) for the rights to genes sequenced by Human Genome Sciences. In March 1994, Hoffman-LaRoche agreed to invest more than $70 million in Millennium Pharmaceuticals for the right to exploit genes relating to obesity and adult-onset diabetes.*

Erramouspe, 1996

In Britain alone, the number of biotech companies grew from 386 in 1994 to 485 in 1995 (House of Commons, Science and Technology Committee, 1995, para. 149). As the founder and chief executive of Sequana Therapeutics, Kevin Kinsella, a veteran venture capitalist said in the early 1990s:

> *As a venture capitalist, I've started seven biotech companies since 1982, but I haven't seen anything like it. This is biotech's counterpart of the Oklahoma land rush.*

Bylinsky, 1994

An article in the British daily newspaper, *The Independent*, reported that one US company, Myriad Genetics, has applied to patent the use of a gene that predisposes women to breast cancer, both for diagnostic tests and for therapeutic treatment. It has plans to start UK marketing for the test which in the US sells for around £1,500 (*The Independent*, June 29, 1997).

In a recent review of the commercialisation of human genetics, Timothy Caulfield concluded:

> . . . *the number of biotechnology companies has grown substantially; the value of stocks in biotech companies continue to soar; large cooperative deals have been struck between emerging genome research companies and established pharmaceutical corporations, there are substantial connections between for-profit clinical genetic diagnostic companies and academic institutions; over 1,175 patents were granted on human genetic sequences between 1981 and 1995; and universities and government research centres are increasingly turning to the private sector for collaborative financial support.*

> Caulfield, 1997

The commercial investment in research and development is based on predictions that profits will ensue from new medications and drugs aimed at specific conditions. Commercial applications of research include on-going attention to the ability to ensure patent protection (Thomas et al, 1996). Firms are investing heavily in finding and cataloguing 'defective' genes and are involved in what has been called 'racing to refine their gene-hunting technology and expand their competitive edge' (Bylinsky, 1994).

The knowledge that genomics is generating is predicted to pay off in a number of ways. Detecting disease ('genetic diagnostics') and gauging its severity is the area in which many genomic start-ups are looking for their first commercial success. (For example, laboratory chips are being developed that combine a chemical test and electronic sensors to test for a specific disease.) Gene therapy (administering replacement genes even in the womb for such conditions as muscular dystrophy, haemophilia, cancer and cystic fibrosis), regulating genes (replacing command sequences), protein therapy (medicinal proteins injected directly into the bloodstream) and the development of genetically derived drugs are other areas of commercial promise that make human genetics big business.

As the head of one of the largest genomics firms (Sequana's Kinsella) confidently stated: 'The payoff of genomics will be bigger than that of the Manhattan Project or the space program' (Bylinsky, 1994). It is big business and big profit from this perspective.

The perspective of the law

From the perspective of law, there are a number of issues that are already beginning to filter their way into the court rooms in many nations. Some are more likely to be problematic depending on the legal and social structure of the particular state, but there is clearly legal wrangling that will ensue and some very real dilemmas raised by the prospect of vast genetic knowledge.

The types of issues that have already reached the courts include issues of knowledge available before birth – abortion, 'wrongful birth' and 'wrongful conception'. Selective abortion has been legalised in a number of countries based on prenatal screening that indicates particular phenotypes (characteristics) – usually those that can be related to some condition that is considered undesirable because it disables. A key question of these types of cases is whether it is better not to be born at all than to be born with a disability and how such a decision could be taken by a third party. Solomon would have been troubled; the courts certainly are.

Other questions that concern legal scholars and courtroom lawyers are privacy and the confidentiality of genetic knowledge. Who owns the knowledge and what are the responsibilities of those who have the information to pass it on to the individual whose genetic information it is? How confidential is the information? To whom should it be given when it involves future generations or public health risks? Issues of informed consent have always provided a legal quagmire but in the case of genetic information, this is compounded because future generations are implicated.

Finally, there are a whole set of issues raised around access to new reproductive technology both in terms of nations being able to access the technology but also the risk that there could be individual or collective cases of discrimination in determining who gets access to which technology.

So genetics provides fertile ground for legal dilemmas that are already before the courts and likely to increase with issues of access, of privacy, and of legal culpability.

The perspective of genetic counselling

The role of genetic counsellors, whether they are geneticists or other medical or health personnel, is to help prospective parents to determine possible options and a course of action with respect to the genetic information available. For the counsellor, the questions that arise are: how to determine which of the genes suggest positive and beneficial outcomes and in which circumstances, and which are negative; and how to provide sufficient information for families to make decisions about which risks they choose to take. The risks of the condition are calculated and information is provided about what are often referred to as genetic anomalies, genetic problems and genetic disadvantage. For the genetic counsellor, the accuracy of the diagnosis is critical to enable an accurate risk analysis and appropriate counselling on both the social and individual impact.

Dilemmas and debates arise among genetic counsellors about which tests are legitimate and which their patients or clients should not be advised to undergo. Some genetic counsellors draw lines in terms of the types of genetic information that are useful for individuals, for families, or for susceptible groups to have. Distinctions are sometimes drawn between the physical characteristics identifiable through genetic tests and the psychological or behavioural characteristics. Questions arise about the legitimacy of some information and the relative contribution of genetic matter in relation to socio-environmental contributors to particular characteristics. What tests, what information to impart, and what advice to give about the consequences are the dilemmas from the perspective of genetic counselling.

The recent emphasis on patient autonomy in health care decision-making underlines the potential tension between the individual's perceived right of access to information and the professional's own moral views on prenatal diagnosis and what ought to be screened for: what ought to be the basis of good professional practice.

The perspective of policy-makers

Policy-makers are raising issues about the outcome and use of the knowledge that results from genetic research and its application. How will public policy take into account the knowledge available and the social issues that are raised by that knowledge? Questions are arising about the interplay between the Human Genome Project and the provision of health care, employment provisions in anti-discrimination law, employment equity law, return to work initiatives (including Workers Compensation legislation), health and safety regulation, insurance policies and the provision of social services.

In February 1997, for example, the Association of British Insurers announced that British people wishing to take out new life insurance policies would have to reveal the results of genetic tests they had undergone, even though they were not required to take tests to qualify for insurance. (Their current guidelines state that members should not ask applicants to take tests, but can require them to disclose the results of any taken in the past; Clark, 2000.) Many US companies require applicants for insurance to undergo genetic testing. The Association of British Insurers in announcing the policy stated:

> *It is important that insurance companies continue to see the results of genetic tests so they can monitor developments and gauge any financial impact on their company.*

Toronto Star, February 19, 1997

One concern is that genetic discrimination occurs when, on the basis of real or perceived differences in their genomes, qualified individuals are denied rights or privileges that are available to others. This can occur in health care, in employment, in insurance policies, in social services and in other areas of public policy. The rapid advances in genetic testing, therapy and technology, have increased the possibility of stigmatisation and discrimination against individuals with current and possible future genetic disorders in many areas of daily life. There are significant implications for public policy but there has been little systematic identification of measures that will need to be in place to deal with the availability of genetic information.

Governments in a number of countries have committed themselves to community living for individuals, equality of employment opportunities, equal access to health care and equity in social services. Central to these policy initiatives are understanding and guidance on how eligibility and qualifications are defined and the type of differentiation that can be used to include and exclude individuals. What are essential qualifications for a job? How are scarce resources in medicine to be distributed? What is the basis for determining the level of service to which an individual will be entitled? What would constitute undue hardship on an employer? What is 'reasonable accommodation' or adjustments or changes to be undertaken by employers or service providers so that disabled people are not disadvantaged in comparison with their non-disabled peers? All of these questions have to be addressed in the light of genetic knowledge.

Let me give an example. It might be said that people with certain genetic disabilities are 'unqualified' for a job if they pose a direct safety or health threat to themselves or others in the workplace. Policy-makers have to ask how likely those risks are. Is a future risk sufficient to exclude a person from a job now? Will this create two further classes of people: those who are employable and those who are not employable – because of genetic characteristics rather than current disability? Can an employer refuse to hire a qualified individual, even though they do not have symptoms of a disease, if occupational exposure to certain substances is likely to increase an employee's known genetic susceptibility to disease?

These are the very real conditions that governments have been trying to address with legislation and policy that prohibits discrimination based on disability and with training and employment initiatives to get people with disabilities into the labour force.

Another area of concern in social policy is the growth of the biotech sector. It is considered good socio-economic policy and an important part of economic development at the present time to encourage the growth of this sector. Any policy that limits this growth, even if implemented for the purposes of protecting consumers of genetic services, or to ensure that anti-discrimination measures are adhered to, tends to meet with resistance. The House of Commons Science and

Technology Committee, for example, in its report on human genetics cautioned that intellectual development and the research infrastructure might fail if they were subject to regulation (House of Commons, 1995).

There were similar arguments about the imperative of freedom of research in genomics, and the consequences that might ensue if that scientific freedom were not protected, during the UNESCO International Bioethics Committee debates on the Declaration of Human Rights and the Human Genome (International Bioethics Committee of UNESCO, 1994, 1995, 1996). The debate then, is whether social policy should try to regulate the biotech industry – and attempt to leash the scientific free-flow – or encourage growth, by minimising regulatory measures aimed at safeguarding consumers (which might inhibit developments).

The perspective of social sciences
The relationship of prenatal screening to attitudes towards people with disabilities has been the subject of a number of social science research studies. If there is a relationship, are attitudes the independent variable or the dependent variable, that is, which influences which? Are all attitudes equally acceptable from a social perspective and how are trade-offs made? Does society tolerate all attitudes or is there some way of deciding what is socially acceptable? Where are the limits? Are there prohibitions in terms of action that people may take, knowing their genetic options? How are social costs and benefits weighed and how does a society tolerate diversity?

Psychologists and others raise another whole host of questions about the anxiety of individuals and the consequences of that anxiety and its implications for genetic testing and screening.

Studies of the genetic basis of intelligence, socio-biology and subcategories such as evolutionary psychology, have engendered a great deal of scientific and social debate. (They led to the eugenics movements of the early part of the twentieth century, which advocated selective breeding to 'improve' human populations.) Controversies around biometric genetic analysis of intellectual abilities were revived with the best-selling book, *The bell curve* (Herrnstein and Murray, 1994) which presented significant differences in IQ between racial groups. The findings of these types of studies and the newly available technology in genetic mapping raises questions about the balance of genes and of environment as contributing factors to differences between people and the immutable nature of genetics (Flanagan et al, 1997).

Moral and ethical questions
The realm of bioethics raises yet another set of questions – questions that address cost and benefit, advantage and disadvantage and the moral ethical standards and principles by which societies operate.

Such questions may be the bread and butter of the bioethicist, but the new genetic research and knowledge impact on the fundamental nature of humanity and give rise to much wider debates on questions like these:

- Do all people have equal moral and social claims?

- What does 'best interests' mean?

- How do we determine the greatest good for the greatest number?

- What is autonomy?

- What is absolute?

- What is risk?

- What is suffering?

There are two underlying elements claimed for the ethics of health care decision-making. One is that there may be certain courses of action that should be ruled out no matter what their presumed benefits; the second is whether the potential good outweighs the possible harm (Nuffield Council on Bioethics, 1993). These may also be the basis for determining the procedural ethics of genetic screening and the use of other gene technology. Consent, confidentiality and the means of measuring benefits and adverse consequences are the ethical dilemmas to be confronted and debated.

There is, however, another set of questions asked by ethicists with respect to the broader social questions about gene research and use of genetic technology and the implications for collective responsibilities. Ethicists in this case are involved in debates about the ethical principles for research and development in the field. (See for example the UNESCO Universal Declaration on the Human Genome and Human Rights, 1997.) Questions are raised about the nature of scientific knowledge and the way in which such knowledge and its associated techniques is used. There is concern with balancing the freedom of research to enable the release of scientific energy that may benefit humankind in both the short term and into the foreseeable future with the risks of eugenic practices or of breaching human rights, both collective and individual.

Inclusion International (formerly the International League of Societies for Persons with a Mental Handicap) is an organisation dedicated to the human rights of people with intellectual disabilities. It has more than 20,000 local associations in over 100 countries representing the estimated 50 million people in the world who have been labelled 'intellectually disabled'. It has adopted a set of guidelines which it sets out as the ethical principles which must be followed in the biotech-nological industry and in genetic practices if the rights of all people are to be protected in the framework of the bio-revolution. The principles are justice (equality of outcome); non-discrimination; human diversity and self-determination and autonomy. The UNESCO Universal Declaration on the Human Genome and Human Rights (October 1997), the European Bioethics Treaty (September 26, 1996) and the International Bar Association all have developed ethical standards for their members in this area (though they do not all share the same emphasis or the same philosophical premises).

The ethics of the biotechnology enterprise itself as well as the procedural ethics in the application of the technology are the important debates of bioethics.

Disability rights advocates and advocates of other groups vulnerable to the implications of the research

For many people in the disability and equality rights movement, genetic research and its application and the identification of genetic anomalies is not so much about science as about the place of difference in society. It raises fundamental issues of the place of disabled people in society and of the potential for discrimination based on genetic characteristics. Discrimination has been a way of life for people with disabilities, and for their families as it has been for aboriginal peoples and for women – all groups who are taking seriously the implications or potential outcomes of the new genetics.

There are fears about the consequences of the rise in 'geneticisation' – the tendency to equate biology with human genetics, to the neglect of the whole host of other social factors that have an impact on the human condition (Lippman, 1991). In its application to people with disabilities, geneticisation has the potential to perpetuate and reinforce the view of disability as a bio-medical abnormality and individual pathology. While there is a biological reality to impairment or disability, the proposition that genetic codes are the primary determinants of what happens within an individual's body does not take account of the influence of the social and environmental conditions that shape people's life circumstances and experiences (Wolfe, 1995). Hence concerns that the rapid increase in genetic knowledge, the rise of geneticisation, the history of eugenics in this century, and the widespread discrimination and negative social attitudes about disability may lead to social pressure for a new eugenics movement. The perception of people with disabilities, and the definition of 'normality', shift with genetic understanding and with the belief that disabled people may be preventable or avoidable through the use of genetic services. The implication is that certain genes are bad or undesirable and should not be passed on to other generations. The idea that it is a positive achievement to eliminate a certain condition changes social perceptions about disability. This has been referred to as 'laissez-faire eugenics'; that is, there are assumptions made about who society 'does not want'.

There are a number of pressures on parents towards selective termination of foetuses with identified genetic characteristics. Social or cultural pressure results from the tendency to portray disability as an 'overwhelming tragedy' in the press; financial pressure comes with the knowledge that disability is costly and can lead to poverty; technological pressure is a factor when there is the knowledge of a condition, and counselling is based on negative views of living with a disability. These kinds of pressures reflect the narrowing notion of the type of diversity and difference that is desirable. They provide the structure of the debates about genetic knowledge and the hesitation to embrace the bio-revolution by those whose vested interests lie in diversity, in difference and in equality rights.

What does it all add up to?

Creating a world view or finding a consensus is not a simple enterprise. Genetic research and its application is not an abstract science – or even a moral one; it is inherently political. Nation states clearly are playing secondary roles in the debate that is going on. There may be some cross-overs between the different parties and perspective involved, but on the whole they have different cultures, each prone to addressing the questions in different ways. Languages are not common and each perspective claims supremacy. Fundamental assumptions about the meaning of humankind are being raised. Critical questions about the proper limits of science are being asked. Important dilemmas are emerging about whose view of the ordered universe will be adopted.

What does the future hold?

In the coming years we will be hearing a lot more about the ethical and social issues arising from genetic research. Hopefully there may be many more discussions and debates about what is acceptable and what is not in terms of tampering with our collectively owned genetic codes. What is at stake here is what we value in our humanness and how we understand the importance of diversity in society. Genetic research, information, screening and testing can be used to promote difference and diversity, to encourage interdependence or it can be used to limit difference, to screen, to create similarity. It is an important choice we have to make – a choice that must be collectively made. It provides a challenge for all the players to find ways to hold the discussions, to share language and ideas, to recognise and respect the many perspectives and interests, and to be wise. The consequence of not being able to meet that challenge is a frightening one.

References

Bylinsky, G. (1994) Genetics: the money rush is on. *Fortune*.

Caulfield, T. (1997) *The commercialization of human genetics: a discussion of issues relevant to the Canadian Consumer*. Draft (August 23). Prepared for Industry Canada, Office of Consumer Affairs.

Clark, A. (2000) Insurance risks. *The Guardian, Special Supplement*, The story of life. The mapping of the human genome, June 26, 11

Cohen, J. (1997) The genomics gamble. 275 *Science* 767.

Erramouspe, M. (1996) Staking claims on the human blueprint: rewards and rent-dissipating races. 43 *UCLA Law Review* 961.

Flanagan, D.P., et al (1997) *Contemporary intellectual assessment*. New York: The Guilford Press.

Gert, B. (1966) A brief history of the Genome Project. In B. Gert et al (eds) *Morality and the new genetics: a guide for students and health care providers*. Sudbury, Massachusetts: Jones and Bartlett Publishers.

Herrnstein, R.J. and Murray, C. (1994) *The bell curve: intelligence and class structure in American life*. New York: Free Press.

House of Commons, Science and Technology Committee (1995) *Third report: human genetics: the science and its consequences*. London: House of Commons, Session 1994–95.

International Bioethics Committee of UNESCO (1994, 1995, 1996) *Proceedings*. Geneva: UNESCO.

Lippman, A. (1991) Prenatal genetic testing and screening: constructing needs and reinforcing inequities. *American Journal of Law and Medicine* 17 (1 & 2): 15–20.

Nuffield Council on Bioethics (1993) *Genetic screening, ethical issues*. London: Nuffield Council on Bioethics.

Somerville, M.A. (1996) Are we just 'gene machines' or also 'secular sacred'? From new science to a new societal paradigm. *Policy Options* 17(2).

Thomas, S.M., et al (1996) Ownership of the human genome. 380 *Nature* 387.

Toronto Star, (1997) February 19.

Toronto Star, (1997) March 13.

UNESCO (1997) *Universal Declaration on the Human Genome and Human Rights.* Geneva: UNESCO.

Wolfe S. M. (1995) Beyond genetic discrimination: toward the broader harm of geneticism. *Journal of Law, Medicine and Ethics* 23: 345–53.

Glossary (Dictionary)

An explanation of words used in this book

In putting together these explanations of medical, scientific and other difficult words, the following books or pamphlets were particularly useful:

Agnes Fletcher (1997) It's not the baby's responsibility to be perfect, *Amazons* (Newsletter of the British Council of Disabled People's Women's Group) June: 1, 4, 5.

Philip Kitcher (1996) *The lives to come: the genetic revolution and human possibilities*. London: Penguin.

Marcus Pembrey (1996) The new genetics: a user's guide. In Teresa Marteau and Martin Richards (eds) *The troubled helix: social and psychological implications of the new human genetics*. Cambridge: Cambridge University Press.

Tracey Sutela and Anita Badami (1997) *The new reproductive technologies: a plain language guide*. Burnaby, British Columbia (Canada): The Lower Mainland Community Based Services Society.

Achondraplasia   A disorder of cartilage formation in the foetus that means the child/adult has restricted growth.

Amniocentesis   Prenatal test that involves removing a small amount of the fluid surrounding a foetus in the womb, using a needle passed through the abdomen with ultrasound guidance. The fluid is analysed for chromosomal abnormalities (eg Down's syndrome) and other conditions (eg spina bifida). Results can take several weeks. (The risk of miscarriage following the amniocentesis is relatively low after the first three months of pregnancy but depends on the skill of the person carrying out the procedure.)

Anomaly or abnormality (eg genetic or chromosomal anomaly or abnormality)   A difference from normal.

Bioethics   Study of the ethical issues raised by medical and scientific research (eg developments in genetics).

Biometry/biometric   The application of statistics to problems in biology; the measurement of living things and the processes associated with life.

Biotechnology   Research and development derived from affecting biological processes (eg genetic research).

Cell   The smallest part of a living being.

Chorion villous sampling   A prenatal test in which a sample is taken from the tissue surrounding the foetus using a needle and ultrasound guidance. Usually carried out between weeks eight and 11 of pregnancy, it has a higher risk of miscarriage than amniocentesis (2–4%) and a greater risk of unclear results. The test enables prenatal diagnosis of congenital disorders like Down's syndrome and thalassaemia (a hereditary blood disease leading to anaemia).

Chromosomes   Thread-like structures in a cell which carry the genes.

Cloning   Technique of making multiple copies of a segment of DNA.

Congenital (**condition**)   A condition that is present in a baby when it is born.

Cystic fibrosis   This is a hereditary condition inherited from both parents (ie the child is affected only if both parents pass on the gene in question). The disease is most common in people from northern Europe. People with cystic fibrosis used to die young from a variety of digestive, respiratory and pancreatic problems but now may live into their forties. It is a condition for which some hold out great hopes of 'gene therapy' (ie replacement of the gene involved with a gene that functions properly).

Diabetes   A condition in which sugars in the body are not processed properly to produce energy because of a lack of insulin (a hormone in the pancreas). There appears to be an inherited tendency to some forms of diabetes; it may be triggered by various factors, including physical stress.

DNA   Short for DeoxyriboNucleic Acid. The genetic material which controls heredity (biological similarities between parents and children). It is found in the cell nucleus.

Dominant gene (see Mendel/mendelian)

Down's syndrome   A condition arising from an additional chromosome (there are three number 21 chromosomes instead of the usual two), which leads to learning difficulties. The condition can be diagnosed prenatally by amniocentesis and chorionic villus sampling.

Eugenics   The science that is concerned with 'improving the human race', traditionally either by increasing the 'best stock' or by hindering marriages and the production of offspring by those seen as being 'unfit'. The Eugenics movement has generally negative connotations within Europe because of its extreme expression in the policies of Nazi Germany.

Foetus   Name given to a baby in the womb from eight weeks until birth.

Fragile X syndrome   Believed to be the most common identifiable cause of inherited learning disability which shows itself in a wide range of difficulties with learning and developmental delay.

Gene therapy   New ways of treating genetic disease which are still under development. Gene therapy aims either to add a gene that works, when one is missing or not having an effect, or to replace a troublesome gene with one that works properly.

Genes   The instructions in cells (the smallest part of a living being) which decide how your body will form and grow. Genes are inherited from parents.

Genetic condition (or disorder)   A condition, disease, impairment or disability caused by genes.

Genetic counselling   Information or advice given by a health professional (the genetic counsellor) to an individual, couple or family about a medical condition or disease that is, or may be, genetic in origin.

Genetic diversity   Variety and difference in genetic makeup. Some genetic differences may have positive functions, many of which may not yet be known. For example, the carrier condition of sickle cell anaemia occurs when the gene in question is inherited from only one parent. This generally causes no symptoms but gives some protection from malaria, which may account for the high frequency of the gene in malarial areas.

Genetic engineering   Ways of interfering with or changing genes; for example, replacing a 'faulty' gene with a working one.

Genetic mapping   Mapping the order of genes along either part of a chromosome, a whole chromosome or several chromosomes.

Genetic mutation   A change in some of the genetic material of a cell.

Geneticisation   Believing that everything about people can be explained by genetics.

Genome   All the genetic material of a cell.

Genomics   The study of the interactions of genes and cells and biochemistry

Haemoglobin   A substance within the red blood cells.

Human Genome Project/Organisation (HUGO)   Project to map all the genetic material in humans.

Huntington's Disease (Chorea)   A hereditary, degenerative disease that usually appears between 30 and 45 years of age. The genetic basis of the disease has been identified but there are no known effective treatments or cures to prevent the (eventually fatal) mental deterioration which results.

In vitro fertilisation   Fertilisation of an egg outside the body. (The fertilised egg is then incubated and implanted in the woman's uterus or womb.)

Mendel/mendelian   Mendel's rules of inheritance showed that inheritance of characteristics was controlled by particles now known as genes. There are three patterns of inheritance:

i   **autosomal dominant inheritance** – this means the condition is inherited from just one parent. An affected individual has a 50:50 chance of passing it on at each pregnancy, no matter who their partner is, eg Huntington's chorea.

ii   **autosomal recessive inheritance** – this is a condition (eg cystic fibrosis or thalassaemia) which is inherited from both parents. The child is affected only if both parents pass on a 'faulty' gene. Often both parents are healthy carriers (they are not affected by the condition themselves but carry it in their genes). They may well not know they face a one in four chance of having an affected baby with any pregnancy.

iii   **X-linked inheritance** – here only boys are affected but the condition (eg haemophilia, fragile X syndrome) can be passed on by women, who may themselves be unaffected and not know they are carriers of it.

Neural tube defects   A group of abnormalities recognised or present at birth caused by a failure of the neural tube (the structure from which the brain and spinal chord develop) to close (eg spina bifida).

New reproductive technologies   Scientific developments in fertilisation, pregnancy and childbirth such as prenatal testing and *in vitro* fertilisation.

Nuchal scan or nuchal translucency test   Measurement of the nuchal fold at the back of the foetus' neck using ultrasound. An especially wide fold can indicate an increased chance of the foetus having Down's syndrome. Usually done after about 11 weeks of pregnancy.

Nucleotides   Part of DNA.

Phenotypes   The observable characteristics of a person which result from their genes (eg eye colour, body build).

Phenylketonuria (PKU)   A condition which affects babies only if both parents are carriers of a particular 'defective' gene. The defect leads to the build up of amino acid (called phenylalanine) in the bloodstream causing damage to the brain. If untreated this leads to severe learning difficulties. Screening new born babies by testing a blood sample means the condition can be detected soon enough for dietary treatment to prevent any brain damage.

Prenatal (diagnostic) testing   Testing the foetus in the mother's womb before it is born (eg amniocentesis, chorion villous sampling).

Recessive gene (see Mendel/mendelian)

Sanfilippo syndrome   A genetic condition which is first noticed between two and five years of age. The child becomes progressively more intellectually disabled and increasingly unsteady. The disease is progressive; it is unusual for those affected to live beyond twenty.

Serum screening   Serum screening is the technical term for blood tests. Since the late 1970s, the measurement of maternal serum alpha feoaprotein (MSAFP) in a mother's blood has been widely used in the UK to screen for neural tube defects. During the late 1980s, as the incidence of neural tube defects was falling and ultrasound was becoming more sensitive and specific, a number of UK hospitals started to abandon mass screening. However, it was then discovered that low levels of MSAFP were associated with Down's syndrome. Since then, there has been a renewed interest in serum screening which is usually carried out at 10–12 weeks, with results generally available within one week. The accuracy of the test depends critically on the age of the foetus being correctly known because the level of MSAFP increases by about

19% per week in the second three months of pregnancy. Women whose serum screening result indicates an increased risk of neural tube defects or Down's syndrome will then be offered a further diagnostic test; usually ultrasound for neural tube defects and amniocentesis for Down's syndrome.

Sickle cell disease A blood disease that mainly affects people of African origins but also occurs in the Mediterranean region, with high frequencies in parts of Saudi Arabia and India. It occurs when the sickle cell gene is inherited from both parents, and is characterised by the production of an abnormal type of haemoglobin (substance within the red blood cells) which causes obstruction of blood vessels and bleeding especially when the person is ill.

Social model of disability The social model of disability recognises that the disadvantages and discrimination experienced by disabled people, including people with learning difficulties, are caused or exacerbated not by the individual's impairment but by attitudes, barriers and systems in a society which has not been organised to meet their needs (for example, lack of wheelchair access to buildings and transport). By contrast, a medical model of disability concentrates primarily on the physical or intellectual impairment of the individual and about curing or caring for that, ie the focus is on rehabilitation and cure rather than on social support, anti-discrimination and human or civil rights for disabled people.

Spina bifida A condition in which a new born baby has part of the spinal chord and its coverings exposed though a gap in the backbone. Spina bifida is associated with abnormally high levels of a substance (called alpha-fetoprotein) in the fluids surrounding the baby in the womb. The condition can be diagnosed at about the sixteenth week of pregnancy by testing the mother's blood and confirmed by amniocentesis.

Thalassaemia A hereditary blood disease, widespread in the Mediterranean countries, Asia and Africa in which abnormal haemoglobin interferes with the functioning of red blood cells, leading to anaemia and other problems. Children inheriting the disease from both parents are severely affected (thalassaemia major) but those inheriting it from only one parent do not usually have any symptoms. People with the major disease are treated with repeated blood transfusions. The disease can be detected in prenatal tests.

Ultrasound scan   An ultrasound scan uses sound waves to get a picture of the foetus while it is in the mother's womb. It can help date a pregnancy and may tell if there is anything unusual about the foetus (as well as if it is a girl or boy or twins). Routine scans are taken at 12 weeks; later scans may be taken to look for abnormalities in the foetus.

Wrongful birth/conception/life   Lawsuits brought against parents by children, or against doctors by parents, when a choice to detect or 'prevent' the birth of a disabled child (eg through prenatal testing and subsequent termination of pregnancy) was not made or offered.

List of contributors

Priscilla Alderson is a researcher at the Social Science Research Unit in London University's Institute of Education. She has researched young people's wisdom and competence, mainly in hospitals and schools. She was the UK partner in a European Commission research programme on prenatal screening (Biomed II contract no. BMH4 CT96 0704) which included interviews with 40 adults who have inherited conditions which are commonly screened for. Other recent work includes a survey of children's rights, a book on research with disabled students in special and integrated schools and a study of ethics and the impact of genetics on perinatal services.

Ruth Chadwick is Head of the Centre for Professional Ethics and Professor of Moral Philosophy, University of Central Lancashire. She is a member of the Ethics Committee of the Human Genome Organisation (HUGO) and was Chair of its Subcommittee on Cloning. She is also a member of the Food Ethics Council (Chair of the Working Party on Novel Foods) and of the National Committee for Philosophy. She has co-ordinated a number of multinational and multidisciplinary research projects on ethical issues in genetics, funded by the European Commission and by the European Parliament. She was Secretary of the International Association of Bioethics 1992–7.

Agnes Fletcher is a disabled writer and activist. She formerly worked for the International Information Network, Disability Awareness in Action and is now Research Assistant to the British All Party Parliamentary Disablement Group and Parliamentary Liaison Officer for RADAR, a national disability organisation.

Joyce Howarth is a freelance training consultant who has been working with people with learning difficulties since 1980. Much of this work has been around sexual health and empowerment.

Sue and John Picton are the parents of a daughter and a son who both have multiple impairments (caused by an undiagnosed, but presumed recessive genetic metabolic error). Their children are both now in their late twenties and had, in 1997, recently moved into a bungalow which was part of an excellent new project run by the Home Farm Trust. Since leaving full-time education both of them have had a very difficult time trying to find supported independent living in the community that met their needs. Now, both are very happy, and settled in their new home.

Marcia Rioux is Policy Adviser to Inclusion International and former President of the Roeher Institute, Canada's national institute for the study of public policy affecting disabled people. Dr Rioux is also the Adjunct Professor of Social Policy in the Faculty of Environmental Studies at York University. She has published over 50 articles and monographs in law, public policy, disability and medical and health journals. She has acted as the Director of Research and been Principal Investigator on studies on poverty, social well being, disability income systems, violence and abuse, and equality and difference. In addition to her lectures and community involvement in Canada, Dr Rioux has represented The Roeher Institute in Europe, the Caribbean, Eastern Europe and Central and South America. She serves on the editorial board of a number of journals including *Abilities* magazine, *Canadian Journal of Rehabilitation, European Journal on Mental Disability*, and the *Tizard Learning Disability Review* journal, and is Vice President of the International Association for the Scientific Study of Intellectual Disability. She also represents Inclusion International on the International Bioethics Committee on the Human Genome Project of UNESCO.

Jackie Rodgers is a Research Fellow at the Norah Fry Research Centre, University of Bristol. She has a particular interest in how people with learning difficulties can be involved in research and can have a voice in all discussions that relate to them.

Oliver Russell trained as a child psychiatrist. He has worked for over 30 years with children and adults with learning disabilities. From 1988 to 2000 he was Honorary Director of the Norah Fry Research Centre. He was a member of the Committee of Enquiry set up by the Mental

Health Foundation to review the future of community care for people with learning disabilities. He chairs the trustees of the British Institute of Learning Disabilities and is also a trustee of Circles Network. He is currently seconded to the Department of Health as Senior Policy Adviser (Learning Disabilities) where he is involved in the Government's strategic review of services for people with learning disabilities and is leader of the health sub-group.

Tom Shakespeare is Research Development Officer at the Policy, Ethics and Life Sciences Research Institute, Newcastle. He has written and broadcast widely on disability and genetics issues, and is co-author of *Genetic Politics: from Eugenics to Genome* (New Clarion Press, forthcoming 2001).

Linda Ward is Director at the Norah Fry Research Centre, University of Bristol; she has researched and written widely in the field of learning difficulties since 1980. She is also Policy and Practice Development Manager (Disability) at the Joseph Rowntree Foundation – the largest independent funder of applied research and innovative development projects in the field of disability, social care and housing in the UK, and was formerly Social Research Adviser to the National Lottery Charities Board's Health, Disability and Care grants programme.

Chapter 3 – 'Difference and choice: a workshop for people with learning difficulties' was written by Joyce Howarth and Jackie Rodgers, with contributions by **Alison Collins, Brenda Cook, Graham Hamblett, Collette Harris, Jackie Long, Zara May and Bruce Webster** from two workshops facilitated by Joyce and Jackie, with support for participants from Katie May, Jennie Mortimore, Jane Sallis and Katherine Stevenson.

Other titles from the
British Institute of Learning Disabilities

Forgotten Lives
Exploring the History of Learning Disability

Edited by Dorothy Atkinson, Mark Jackson and Jan Walmsley

"This book is so informative, funny and moving that I cannot imagine anyone not liking it or learning something from it."
Nursing Times

This book explores a long-neglected topic: the history of people with a learning disability. *Forgotten Lives* draws on a variety of different perspectives, including first hand accounts from people with a learning disability, documentary evidence, photographs and archive sources.

Staff, service users, and anyone wishing to undertake their own historical research will find it an invaluable resource.

1997   ISBN 1 873971 84 4   £18.95

Caring for Kathleen: A Sister's Story

Margaret Fray

"This book deserves to be read by anyone (including student nurses) who has an interest in caring for people with a learning disability."
Learning Disability Practice

This is Margaret Fray's moving account of her sister Kathleen, who was born with Down syndrome. Kathleen's life reflects the changing shape of services over the past 70 years and the huge gap in provision for people with a learning disability who develop dementia.

Caring for Kathleen provides a vivid description of Margaret's life as a companion and a carer for Kathleen, and is illustrated throughout with pictures from the family album.

2000   ISBN 1 902519 19 1   £15.00

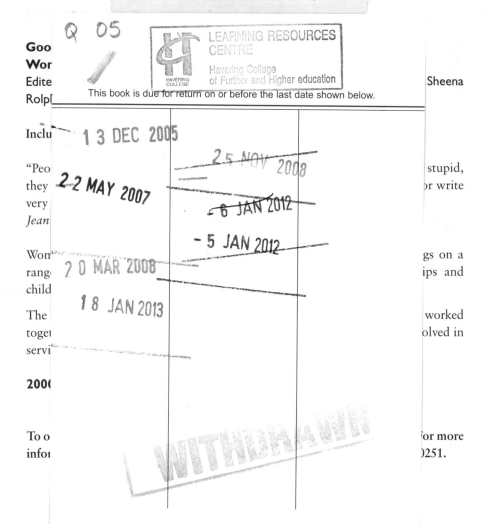

Goo
Wor
Edite   Sheena
Rolpl

Inclu

"Peo   stupid,
they   or write
very
Jean

Won   gs on a
rang   ips and
child

The   worked
toget   olved in
servi

2000

To o   or more
infoi   )251.

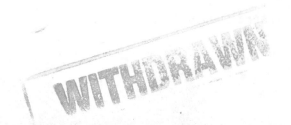